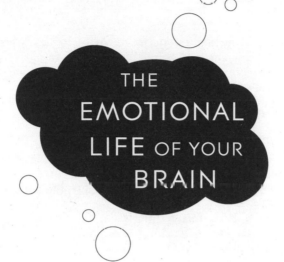

THE
EMOTIONAL
LIFE OF YOUR
BRAIN

'Look forward to cultivating keener attention, having more attunement to others, and being more connected to your own intuition. It's all possible – and this book shows you how.'

Deepak Chopra

'Whether he is measuring neural activity in the laboratory or climbing the Himalayas to meet the Dalai Lama, Davidson is an inveterate explorer who has spent a lifetime probing the deep mystery of human feeling. Don't miss this smart and lively book by the world's foremost expert on emotion and the brain.'

Daniel Gilbert, Ph.D., author of Stumbling on Happiness

'What a gift from the world's leading neuroscientist who works on what makes life worth living. This is a must read for everyone who is interested in positive psychology.'

Martin E. P. Seligman, author of Learned Optimism *and* Flourish

'This superb book is many things – a crystal clear tour of the neuroscience of emotion; a primer about how the scientific process works; a personal story by a really likeable guy; and the promise of a better world. This is a wonderful book.'

Robert M. Sapolsky, Ph.D., author of Why Zebras Don't Get Ulcers

'Richard Davidson, a visionary neuropsychologist, joins with Sharon Begley, one of the most astute science writers, to illuminate the dimensions of our emotional make up and offer cogent and compelling ways for us to grow into more effective and fulfilled selves.'

Jerome Groopman, co-author of Your Medical Mind

'In this spine-tingling journey through the hills of the Himalayas and the circuitry of your brain, visionary neuroscientist Richard Davidson uncovers deep and practical insights into humanity's oldest questions. Who are we as individuals? What are the origins of our minds? How do we find peace and cultivate greater kindness for all? Weaving together the latest neuroscience of brain plasticity and emotion and the timeless wisdom of Buddhist thought, *The Emotional Life of Your Brain* will lead you to answers to these questions, and leave you inspired by science and the promise of change for the better.'

Dacher Keltner, Ph.D., author of Born to Be Good

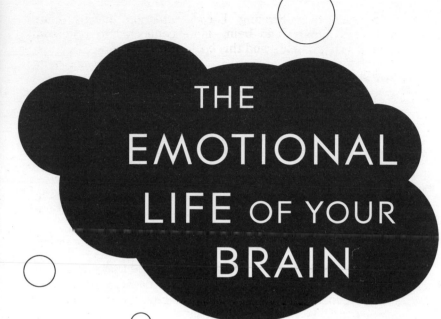

THE
EMOTIONAL
LIFE OF YOUR
BRAIN

HOW ITS UNIQUE PATTERNS AFFECT THE WAY YOU THINK, FEEL, AND LIVE -- AND HOW YOU CAN CHANGE THEM

RICHARD J. DAVIDSON Ph.D.
with **SHARON BEGLEY**

HODDER &
STOUGHTON

PUBLISHER'S NOTE

Every effort has been made to ensure that the information contained in this book is complete and accurate. However, neither the publisher nor the authors can offer specific professional advice or liability to the individual reader. The ideas and suggestions contained in this book are not intended as a substitute for individual medical advice from your health care professional. The authors and the publishers shall not be liable or responsible for any loss or damage allegedly arising from any information or suggestions in this book.

While the author has made every effort to provide accurate telephone numbers and Internet addresses at the time of publication, neither the publisher nor the author assumes any responsibility for errors, or for changes that occur after publication. Further, the publisher does not have any control over and does not assume any responsibility for author or third-party websites or their content.

First published in Great Britain in 2012 by Hodder & Stoughton
An Hachette UK company

First published in the United States of American in 2012 by Hudson Street Press, a member of Penguin Group (USA) Inc.

1

A CIP catalogue record for this title is available from the British Library

ISBN 978 1 444 70880 6
eBook ISBN 978 1 444 70883 7

Printed and bound by Clays Ltd, St Ives plc

Hodder & Stoughton policy is to use papers that are natural, renewable and recyclable products and made from wood grown in sustainable forests. The logging and manufacturing processes are expected to conform to the environmental regulations of the country of origin.

Hodder & Stoughton Ltd
338 Euston Road
London NW1 3BH

www.hodder.co.uk

To Susan, Amelie, and Seth for the love,
grounding, and endless teachings you provide

CONTENTS

INTRODUCTION

A Scientific Quest

This book describes a personal and professional journey to understand why and how people differ in their emotional responses to what life throws at them, motivated by my desire to help people lead healthier, more fulfilling lives. The "professional" thread in this tapestry describes the development of the hybrid discipline called affective neuroscience, the study of the brain mechanisms that underlie our emotions and the search for ways to enhance people's sense of well-being and promote positive qualities of mind. The "personal" thread is my own story. Spurred by the conviction that, as Hamlet said to Horatio, "there are more things in heaven and earth than are dreamt of" in the standard account of the mind provided by mainstream psychology and neuroscience, I have ventured outside the boundaries enclosing these disciplines, sometimes getting struck down, but in the end, I hope, achieving at least some of what I set out to do: to show through rigorous research that emotions, far from being the neurological fluff that mainstream science once believed them to be, are central to the functions of the brain and to the life of the mind.

My thirty years of research in affective neuroscience has produced hundreds of findings, from the brain mechanisms that underlie empathy and the differences between the autistic brain and the normally developing brain to how the brain's seat of rationality can plunge us into the roiling emotional depths of depression. I hope that these results have contributed to our understanding of what it means to be human, of what it means to have an emotional life. But as these findings accumulated, I found myself stepping back from the day-to-day life of my laboratory at the University of Wisconsin, Madison, which has grown over the years to something resembling a small company: As I write this in the spring of 2011, I have eleven graduate students, ten postdoctoral fellows, four computer programmers, twenty-one additional research and administrative staff members, and some twenty million dollars in research grants from the National Institutes of Health and other funders.

Since May 2010, I have also served as director of the university's Center for Investigating Healthy Minds, a research complex dedicated to learning how the qualities of mind that humankind has valued since before the dawn of civilization—compassion, well-being, charity, altruism, kindness, love, and other noble aspects of the human condition—arise in the brain and how they can be nurtured. One of the great virtues of the center is that we do not confine our work to research alone. We very much want to get the results of that research out into the world, where it can make a real difference in the lives of real people. To that end, we have developed a preschool and elementary school curriculum designed to cultivate kindness and mindfulness, and we are evaluating the impact of this training on academic achievement as well as on attention, empathy, and cooperation. Another project investigates whether training in breathing and meditation can help veterans returning from Afghanistan and Iraq cope with stress and anxiety.

I love all of this, both the basic science and the extension of our findings into the real world. But it is way too easy to get consumed by it. (I often joke that I have several full-time jobs, from overseeing grant applications to negotiating with the university bioethics committees for permission to do research on human volunteers.) I did not want that to happen.

About ten years ago, I therefore began to take stock of my research and that of other labs pursuing affective neuroscience—not the interesting individual findings but the larger picture. And I saw that our decades of work had revealed something fundamental about the emotional life of the brain: that each of us is characterized by what I have come to call Emotional Style.

Before I briefly describe the components of Emotional Style, let me quickly explain how it relates to other classification systems that try to illuminate the vast diversity of ways to be human: emotional states, emotional traits, personality, and temperament.

The smallest, most fleeting unit of emotion is an emotional *state*. Typically lasting only a few seconds, it tends to be triggered by an experience the spike of joy you feel at the macaroni collage your child made you for Mother's Day, the sense of accomplishment you feel upon finishing a big project at work, the anger you feel over having to work all three days of a holiday weekend, the sadness you feel when your child is the only one in her class not invited to a party. Emotional states can also arise from purely mental activity, such as daydreaming, or introspection, or anticipating the future. But whether they are triggered by real-world experiences or mental ones, emotional states tend to dissipate, each giving way to the next.

A feeling that does persist, and that remains consistent over minutes or hours or even days, is a *mood*, of the "he's in a bad mood" variety. And a feeling that characterizes you not for days but for years is an emotional *trait*. We think of someone who seems perpetually annoyed as grumpy, and someone who always seems to be mad at the world as angry. An emotional trait (chronic, just-about-to-boil-over anger) increases the likelihood that you will experience a particular emotional state (fury) because it lowers the threshold needed to feel such an emotional state.

Emotional *Style* is a consistent way of responding to the experiences of our lives. It is governed by specific, identifiable brain circuits and can be measured using objective laboratory methods. Emotional Style influences the likelihood of feeling particular emotional states, traits, and moods. Because Emotional Styles are much closer to underlying brain systems than emotional states or traits, they can be considered the atoms of our emotional lives—their fundamental building blocks.

In contrast, personality, a more familiar way of describing people, is neither fundamental in this sense nor grounded in identifiable neurological mechanisms. Personality consists of a set of high-level qualities that comprise particular emotional traits and Emotional Styles. Take, for instance, the well-studied personality trait of *agreeableness*. People who are extremely agreeable, as measured by standard psychological assessments (as well as their own and that of people who know them well), are empathic, considerate, friendly, generous, and helpful. But each of these emotional traits is itself the product of different aspects of Emotional Style. Unlike personality, Emotional Style can be traced to a specific, characteristic brain signature. To understand the brain basis of agreeableness, then, we need to probe more deeply into the underlying Emotional Styles that comprise it.

Psychology has been churning out classification schemes with gusto lately, asserting that there are four kinds of temperament or five components of personality or Lord-knows-how-many character types. While perfectly interesting and even fun—the popular media have had a field day describing which character types make good romantic matches, business leaders, or psychopaths—these schemes are light on scientific validity because they are not based on any rigorous analysis of underlying brain mechanisms. Anything having to do with human behavior, feelings, and ways of thinking arises from the brain, so any valid classification scheme must also be based on the brain. Which brings me back to Emotional Style.

Emotional Style comprises six dimensions. Neither conventional aspects of personality nor simple emotional traits or moods, let alone diagnostic criteria for mental illness, these six dimensions reflect the discoveries of modern neuroscientific research:

- Resilience: how slowly or quickly you recover from adversity.
- Outlook: how long you are able to sustain positive emotion.
- Social Intuition: how adept you are at picking up social signals from the people around you.
- Self-Awareness: how well you perceive bodily feelings that reflect emotions.
- Sensitivity to Context: how good you are at regulating your emotional responses to take into account the context you find yourself in.
- Attention: how sharp and clear your focus is.

These are probably not the six dimensions you would come up with if you sat down and thought about your emotions and how they might differ from those of others. By the same measure, the Bohr model of the atom is probably not the model you would come up with if you sat down and thought about the structure of matter. I don't mean to equate my work with that of the founders of modern physics, only to make a general point: It is rare that the human mind can determine the truths of nature, or even of ourselves, by intuition or casual observation. That's why we have science. Only by methodical, rigorous experiments, and lots of them, can we figure out how the world works—and how we ourselves work.

These six dimensions arose from my research in affective neuroscience, complemented and strengthened by the discoveries of colleagues around the world. They reflect properties of and patterns in the brain, the sine qua non of any model of human behavior and emotion. If the six dimensions don't resonate with your understanding of yourself or of those close to you, that is likely because several of them operate on levels that are not always immediately apparent. For example, we tend not to be consciously aware of where we fall on the Resilience dimension. With few exceptions, we do not pay attention to how quickly we recover from a stressful event. (An exception would be something extremely traumatic, such as the death of a child; in that case, you are all too aware that you have remained a basket case for months and months.) But we experience its consequences. For instance, if you have an argument with your significant other in the morning, you might feel irritable for the entire day—yet not realize that the reason you are snappish and grouchy and churlish is that you have not regained your emotional equilibrium, which is the mark of the Slow to Recover style. I will show you in chapter 3 how you can become more aware of your Emotional Styles, which is the first and most important step in any attempt to either gracefully accept who you are or transform it.

A rule of thumb in science is that any new theory that hopes to supplant what came before must explain the same phenomena that the old theory did, as well as new ones. In order to be accepted as a more accurate and all-encompassing theory of gravity than what Isaac Newton had proposed after he saw the apple fall from the tree (or not), Einstein's general theory of relativity had to explain all of the gravitational phenomena that Newton's did, such as the orbits of the planets around the sun and the rate at which objects fell to earth, and new ones, too, such as the bending of celestial light around a large star. Let me show, then, that Emotional Style has sufficient explanatory power to account for well-established personality traits and temperament types; later, particularly in chapter 4, we will see that it has a solid foundation in the brain, something other classification schemes do not.

I believe that every individual personality and temperament reflects a different combination of the six dimensions of Emotional Style. Take the "big five" personality traits, one of the standard classification systems in psychology: openness to new experience, conscientiousness, extraversion, agreeableness, and neuroticism:

- Someone high in openness to new experience has strong Social Intuition. She is also very self-aware and tends to be focused in her Attention style.
- A conscientious person has well-developed Social Intuition, a focused style of Attention, and acute Sensitivity to Context.
- An extraverted person bounces back rapidly from adversity and thus is at the Fast to Recover end of the Resilience spectrum. She maintains a positive Outlook.
- An agreeable person has a highly attuned Sensitivity to Context and strong Resilience; he also tends to maintain a positive Outlook.
- Someone high in neuroticism is slow to recover from adversity. He has a gloomy, negative Outlook, is relatively insensitive to context, and tends to be unfocused in his Attention style.

While the combinations of Emotional Styles that add up to each of the big five personality traits generally hold true, there will always be exceptions. Not everyone with a given personality will have all the dimensions of Emotional Style that I describe, but they will invariably have at least one of them.

Moving beyond the Big Five, we can look at traits that all of us think of when we describe ourselves or someone we know well. Each of these, too, can be understood as a combination of different dimensions of Emotional Style, though, again, not everyone with the trait will possess each dimension. However, most people will have most of them:

- Impulsive: a combination of unfocused Attention and low Self-Awareness.
- Patient: a combination of high Self-Awareness and high Sensitivity to Context. Knowing that when context changes, other things will change, too, helps to facilitate patience.

- Shy: a combination of being Slow to Recover on the Resilience dimension and having low Sensitivity to Context. As a result of the insensitivity to context, shyness and wariness extend beyond contexts in which they might be normal.
- Anxious: a combination of being Slow to Recover, having a negative Outlook, having high levels of Self-Awareness, and being unfocused (Attention).
- Optimistic: a combination of being Fast to Recover and having a positive Outlook.
- Chronically unhappy: a combination of being Slow to Recover and having a negative Outlook, with the result that a person cannot sustain positive emotions and becomes mired in negative ones after setbacks.

As you can see, these common trait descriptors comprise different permutations of Emotional Styles. This formulation provides a way of describing what the brain bases for these common traits are likely to be.

If you read original scientific papers, it is easy to get the impression that the researchers thought of a question, designed a clever experiment to answer it, and carried out the study with nary a dead end or setback between them and the answer. It's not like that. I suspect you realized as much, but what is not as widely known, even among people who gobble up popular accounts of scientific research, is how difficult it is to challenge a prevailing paradigm. That was the position I found myself in during the early 1980s. At that time, academic psychology relegated the study of emotions mostly to social and personality psychology rather than to neurobiology; few psychology researchers were interested in studying the brain basis of emotion. What little interest there was supported research on the so-called emotion centers of the brain, which were then thought to be exclusively in the limbic system. I had a very different idea: that higher cortical functions, particularly those located in the evolutionarily advanced prefrontal cortex, are critical to emotion.

When I first suggested that the prefrontal cortex is involved in emotion, I was met with an endless stream of skeptics. The prefrontal cortex, they insisted, is the site of reason, the antithesis of emotion. It certainly could not play a role in emotion, too. It was very lonely trying to carve out a scientific career when the prevailing winds blew strongly in the other direction. My search for bases of emotion in the brain's seat of reason was viewed as quixotic, to say the least—the neuroscientific equivalent of hunting elephants in Alaska. There were more than a few times, especially when I struggled to get funding early on, when my skepticism about the classic division between thought (in the highly evolved neocortex) and feeling (in the subcortical limbic system) seemed like a good way to end a scientific career, not begin one.

If my scientific leanings were a less than savvy career move, so were some of my personal interests. Soon after I entered graduate school at Harvard in the 1970s, I met a remarkable group of kind and compassionate people who, I soon learned, had something in common: They all practiced meditation. This discovery catalyzed my then-rudimentary interest in meditation to such an extent that, after my second year of grad school, I went off to India and Sri Lanka for three months to learn more about this ancient tradition and experience what intensive meditation might bring. I had a second motive as well—I wanted to see whether meditation might be a suitable subject for scientific research.

Studying emotions was controversial enough. Practicing meditation was practically heretical, and studying it was a scientific nonstarter. Just as academic psychologists and neuroscientists believed that there are brain regions for reason and brain regions for emotions, and never the two shall meet, so they believed that there is rigorous, empirical science and there is woo-woo meditation—and if you practiced the latter, your bona fides for the former were highly suspect.

This was the period of *The Tao of Physics* (1975), *The Dancing Wu Li Masters* (1979), and other books arguing that there are strong complementarities between the findings of modern Western science and the insights of ancient Eastern philosophies. Most academic scientists dismissed this as trash; being a meditator in their midst was not, shall we say, the most direct path to academic success. It was made very clear to me by my Harvard mentors that if I wanted a successful scientific career, studying meditation was not a very good place to start. While I dabbled in research on meditation in the early part of my career, once I saw how deep the resistance was, I set it aside. I remained a closet meditator, though, and eventually—once I had been granted tenure at the University of Wisconsin, and had a long list of scientific publications and honors to my credit—returned to meditation as a subject of scientific study.

A big reason I did so was a transformative meeting I had with the Dalai Lama in 1992, which completely changed the course of both my career and my personal life. As I describe in chapter 9, the encounter was the spark that made me decide to bring my interests in meditation and other forms of mental training out of the closet.

It is breathtaking to see how much has changed in the short period of time that I've been at this. In less than twenty years, the scientific and medical communities have become much more receptive to research on mental training. Thousands of new articles are now published on the subject in top scientific journals each year (I was tickled that the first such paper ever to appear in the august *Proceedings of the National Academy of Sciences* was by my colleagues and me, in 2004), and the National Institutes of Health now provides substantial funding for research on meditation. A decade ago that would have been unthinkable.

I believe this change is a very good thing, and not because of any sense of personal vindication (though I admit it's been gratifying to see a scientific outcast of a topic receive the respect it deserves). I made two promises to the Dalai Lama in 1992: I would personally study meditation, and I would try to make research on positive emotions, such as compassion and well-being, as central a focus of psychology as research on negative emotions had long been.

Now those two promises have converged, and with them my tilting-at-windmills conviction that the seat of reason and higher-order cognitive function in the brain plays as important a role in emotion as the limbic system does. My research on meditators has shown that mental training can alter patterns of activity in the brain to strengthen empathy, compassion, optimism, and a sense of well-being—the culmination of my promise to study meditation as well as positive emotions. And my research in the mainstream of affective neuroscience has shown that it is these sites of higher-order reasoning that hold the key to altering these patterns of brain activity.

So while this book is a story of my personal and scientific transformation, I hope it offers you a guide for your own transformation. In Sanskrit,

the word for *meditation* also means "familiarization." Becoming more familiar with your Emotional Style is the first and most important step in transforming it. If this book does nothing more than increase your awareness of
your own Emotional Style and that of others around you, I would consider it
a success.

THE
EMOTIONAL
LIFE OF YOUR
BRAIN

CHAPTER 1

■ ■ ■

One Brain Does Not Fit All

If you believe most self-help books, pop-psychology articles, and television therapists, then you probably assume that how people respond to significant life events is pretty predictable. Most of us, according to the "experts," are affected in just about the same way by a given experience—there is *a* grieving process that everyone goes through, there is *a* sequence of events that happens when we fall in love, there is *a* standard response to being jilted, and there are fairly standard ways almost every normal person reacts to the birth of a child, to being unappreciated at one's job, to having an unbearable workload, to the challenges of raising teenagers, and to the inevitable changes that occur with aging. These same experts confidently recommend steps we can all take to regain our emotional footing, weather a setback in life or in love, become more (or less) sensitive, handle anxiety with aplomb . . . and otherwise become the kind of people we would like to be.

But my thirty-plus years of research have shown that these one-size-fits-all assumptions are even less valid in the realm of emotion than they are in medicine. There, scientists are discovering that people's DNA shapes how they will respond to prescription drugs (among other things), ushering in an age of personalized medicine in which the treatments one patient receives for a certain illness will be different from what another patient receives for that same illness—for the fundamental reason that no two patients' genes are identical.

(One important example of this: The amount of the blood thinner warfarin a patient can safely take to prevent blood clots depends on how quickly the patient's genes metabolize the drug.) When it comes to how people respond to what life throws at them, and how they can develop and nurture their capacity to feel joy, to form loving relationships, to withstand setbacks, and in general to lead a meaningful life, the prescription must be just as personalized. In this case, the reason is not just that our DNA differs—though of course it does, and DNA definitely influences our emotional traits—but that our patterns of brain activity do. Just as the medicine of tomorrow will be shaped by deciphering patients' DNA, so the psychology of today can be shaped by understanding the characteristic patterns of brain activity underlying the emotional traits and states that define each of us.

Over the course of my career as a neuroscientist, I've seen thousands of people who share similar backgrounds respond in dramatically different ways to the same life event. Some are resilient in the face of stress, for instance, while others fall apart. The latter become anxious, depressed, or unable to function when they encounter adversity. Resilient people are somehow able not only to withstand but to benefit from certain kinds of stressful events and to turn adversity into advantage. This, in a nutshell, is the puzzle that has driven my research. I've wanted to know what determines how someone reacts to a divorce, to the death of a loved one, to the loss of a job, or to any other setback—and, equally, what determines how people react to a career triumph, to winning the heart of their true love, to realizing that a friend will walk over hot coals for them, or to other sources of happiness. Why and how do people differ so widely in their emotional responses to the ups and the downs of life?

The answer that has emerged from my own work is that different people have different Emotional Styles. These are constellations of emotional reactions and coping responses that differ in kind, intensity, and duration. Just as each person has a unique fingerprint and a unique face, each of us has a unique emotional profile, one that is so much a part of who we are that those who know us well can often predict how we will respond to an emotional challenge. My own Emotional Style, for instance, is fairly optimistic and upbeat, eager to take on challenges, quick to recover from adversity, but sometimes prone to worry about things that are beyond my control. (My mother, struck by my sunny disposition, used to call me her "joy boy.") Emotional Style is why one person recovers fairly quickly from a painful divorce while another remains mired in self-recrimination and despair. It is why one sibling bounces back from a job loss while another feels worthless for years afterward. It is why one father shrugs off the botched call of a Little League umpire who called out his (clearly safe!) daughter at second base while another leaps out of his seat and screams at the ump until his face turns purple. Emotional Style is why one friend serves as a wellspring of solace to everyone in her circle while another makes herself scarce—emotionally and literally—whenever her friends or family need sympathy and support. It is why some people can read body language and tone of voice as clearly as a billboard while to others these nonverbal cues are a foreign language. And it is why some people have insight into their own states of mind, heart, and body that others do not even realize is possible.

Every day presents countless opportunities to observe Emotional Styles in action. I spend a lot of time at airports, and it is a rare trip that doesn't offer the chance for a little field research. As we all know, there seem to be more ways for a flight schedule to go awry than there are flights departing O'Hare on a Friday evening: bad weather, waiting for a flight crew whose connection is late, mechanical problems, cockpit warning lights that no one can decipher . . . the list goes on. So I've had countless chances to watch the reaction of passengers (as well as myself!) who, waiting to take off, hear the dreaded announcement that the flight has been delayed for one hour, or for two hours, or indefinitely, or canceled. The collective groan is audible. But if you look carefully at individual passengers, you'll see a wide range of emotional reactions. There's the college student in his hoodie, bobbing his head to the music coming in through his earbuds, who barely glances up before getting lost again in his iPad. There's the young mother traveling alone with a squirmy toddler who mutters, "Oh great," before grabbing her child and stalking off toward the food court. There's the corporate-looking woman in the tailored suit who briskly walks up to the gate agent and calmly but firmly demands to be rerouted immediately through anywhere this side of Kathmandu—just get her to her meeting! There's the silver-haired, bespoke-suited man who storms up to the agent and, loud enough for everyone to hear, demands to know if she realizes how important it is for him to get to his destination, insists on seeing her superior, and—red-faced by now—screams that the situation is completely intolerable.

Okay, I'm prepared to believe that delays are worse for some people than for others. Failing to make it to the bedside of your dying mother is definitely up there, and missing a business meeting that means life or death to the company your grandfather founded is a lot worse than a student arriving home for winter break half a day later than planned. But I strongly suspect that the differences in how people react to an exasperating flight delay have less to do with the external circumstances and more to do with their Emotional Style.

The existence of Emotional Style raises a number of related questions. The most obvious is, when does Emotional Style first appear—in early adulthood, when we settle into the patterns that describe the people we will be, or, as genetic determinists would have it, before birth? Do these patterns of emotional response remain constant and stable throughout our lives? A less obvious question, but one that arose in the course of my research, is whether Emotional Style influences physical health. (One reason to suspect it does is that people who suffer from clinical depression are much more prone to certain physical disorders such as heart attack and asthma than are people with no history of depression.) Perhaps most fundamentally, how does the brain produce the different Emotional Styles—and are they hardwired into our neural circuitry, or is there anything we can do to change them and thus alter how we deal with and respond to the pleasures and vicissitudes of life? And if we are able to somehow change our Emotional Style (in chapter 11 I will suggest some methods for doing so), does it also produce measureable changes in the brain?

The Six Dimensions

So as not to leave you in suspense—and to make specific what I mean by "Emotional Style"—let me lay out its bare bones. There are six dimensions of Emotional Style. The existence of the six did not just suddenly occur to me, nor did they emerge early on in my research, let alone result from a command decision that six would be a nice number. Instead, they arose from systematic studies of the neural bases of emotion. Each of the six dimensions has a specific, identifiable neural signature—a good indication that they are real and not merely a theoretical construct. It is conceivable that there are more than six dimensions, but it's unlikely: The major emotion circuits in the brain are now well understood, and if we believe that the only aspects of emotion that have scientific validity are those that can be traced to events in the brain, then six dimensions completely describe Emotional Style.

Each dimension describes a continuum. Some people fall at one or the other extreme of that continuum, while others fall somewhere in the middle. The combination of where you fall on each dimension adds up to your overall Emotional Style.

Your Resilience style: Can you usually shake off setbacks, or do you suffer a meltdown? When faced with an emotional or other challenge, can you muster the tenacity and determination to soldier on, or do you feel so helpless that you simply surrender? If you have an argument with your significant other, does it cast a pall on the remainder of your day, or are you able to recover quickly and put it behind you? When you're knocked back on your heels, do you bounce back and throw yourself into the ring of life again, or do you melt into a puddle of depression and resignation? Do you respond to setbacks with energy and determination, or do you give up? People at one extreme of this dimension are Fast to Recover from adversity; those at the other extreme are Slow to Recover, crippled by adversity.

Your Outlook style: Do you seldom let emotional clouds darken your sunny outlook on life? Do you maintain a high level of energy and engagement even when things don't go your way? Or do you tend toward cynicism and pessimism, struggling to see anything positive? People at one extreme of the Outlook spectrum can be described as Positive types; those at the other, as Negative.

Your Social Intuition style: Can you read people's body language and tone of voice like a book, inferring whether they want to talk or be alone, whether they are stressed to the breaking point or feeling mellow? Or are you puzzled by—even blind to—the outward indications of people's mental and emotional states? Those at one extreme on this spectrum are Socially Intuitive types; those at the other, Puzzled.

Your Self-Awareness style: Are you aware of your own thoughts and feelings and attuned to the messages your body sends you? Or do you act and react without knowing why you do what you do, because your inner self is opaque to your conscious mind? Do those closest to you ask why you never engage in introspection and wonder why you seem oblivious to the fact that you are anxious, jealous, impatient, or threatened? At one extreme of this spectrum are people who are Self-Aware; at the other, those who are Self-Opaque.

Your Sensitivity to Context style: Are you able to pick up the conventional rules of social interaction so that you do not tell your boss the same dirty joke you told your husband or try to pick up a date at a funeral? Or are you baffled when people tell you that your behavior is inappropriate? If you are at one extreme of the Sensitivity to Context style, you are Tuned In; at the other end, Tuned Out.

Your Attention style: Can you screen out emotional or other distractions and stay focused? Are you so caught up in your video game that you don't notice the dog whining to go out, until he makes a mess on the floor? Or do your thoughts flit from the task at hand to the fight you had with your spouse this morning or the anxiety you feel about an upcoming presentation for work? At one extreme on the Attention spectrum are people with a Focused style; at the other, those who are Unfocused.

Everyone has elements of each of these dimensions of Emotional Style. Think of the six dimensions as ingredients in the recipe for your emotional makeup. You might have a big dollop of Focused attentional style, a pinch of being Tuned In, and not quite as much Self-Awareness as you'd like. You might have such a Positive Outlook that it overshadows everything else about you, although your lack of Resilience and Puzzlement in social situations often come through. Who you are emotionally is the product of different amounts of each of these six components. Because there are so many ways to combine the six dimensions, there are countless Emotional Styles; everyone's is unique.

Outliers

I discovered the six dimensions of Emotional Style serendipitously, in the course of my research on affective neuroscience, the study of the brain basis of human emotion. I never sat down one day and decided that I would dream up different Emotional Styles and then go do the research that showed they exist. Instead, from early in my career, as I'll explain more fully in the next chapter, I've been fascinated by the existence of individual differences.

Even if you are a careful and habitual reader of science stories, especially those about psychology and neuroscience, you probably don't notice that the conclusion reached by almost every study applies only on average, or to most of the research subjects. Maybe the study found that too many choices impede decision making, or that people base ethical judgments on emotional grounds rather than rational ones; maybe it concluded that when people wash their hands they feel less uncomfortable about committing an unethical act or thinking an immoral thought, or that people tend to prefer the taller political candidate to the shorter one. What you seldom read is that the average response integrates a large range of responses, just as the "average weight" of the adults in your neighborhood does. Reporting and focusing on only that average runs the risk of ignoring some very interesting phenomena, namely, the extremes—in this simple example, people who are dangerously overweight and people who are anorexic, whose existence you would not even suspect if you saw only that the average weight is, say, 175 pounds.

So it is with psychological behavior and emotional responses. There are almost always outliers—the person who does *not* judge members of his own ethnic or national group more charitably than he judges people who are different from him, or the person who does *not* follow the order to administer an electric shock to someone behind a screen in order to help him "learn better." I've always been drawn to the outliers, convinced that research about human behavior, thought, and emotion needs to grapple with individual differences. More than that, I concluded long ago, the fact of individual differences is *the* most salient characteristic of emotion.

That was driven home for me early on. My epiphany came with the chance discovery that people differ by a factor of thirty in the level of activity in their prefrontal cortex—activity associated with happiness and approach or with fear, disgust, anxiety, and withdrawal. From then on, my research focused on individual differences, which led me to the concept of Emotional Style and the dimensions that constitute it.

Each of us responds differently to emotional triggers, and to talk about "most people" or "the average person" completely misses the mark. Understanding the nature of this variation, I felt, would enable each of us to follow the classical imperative "Know thyself."

And it would have other real-world consequences as well. Studying variation in emotional response would allow us to predict who might be vulnerable to mental illness or even a level of anxiety and sadness that falls short of clinical illness, and who would be resilient in the face of adversity.

Mind from Brain

Crucially, each dimension of Emotional Style is grounded in a particular pattern of brain activity. Brain imaging shows that these dimensions were not plucked out of the air. Rather, they reflect measurable, biological activity in, especially, the cortex and the limbic system, shown in the diagram below:

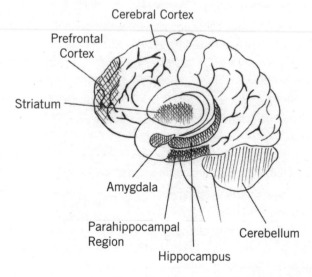

Although the limbic system—including the amygdala and the striatum—was long thought to be the brain's seat of emotion, in fact the cortex also determines our emotional states and moods.

Understanding the neural underpinnings of the six dimensions of Emotional Style, I believe, can empower you to recognize your own overall Emotional Style. Those brain patterns will be the focus of chapter 4, but let me give a preview here. A region of the visual cortex, the large chunk of neural real estate at the back of the brain, seems to be specialized for identifying particular individuals of a group (human or not) in which you have expertise. So, for instance, it becomes active when a classic-car collector scrutinizes a 1952 Nash Healey and a 1963 Shelby Cobra—or when a person studies a face, since we are all experts in faces. (In fact, this fusiform gyrus was originally called the fusiform face area because scientists thought it processed only faces, rather than any exemplars in a person's domain of expertise.) It turns out that people who are unable to sense others' emotions—such as children who fall on the autism spectrum as well as others who are at the Puzzled end of the Social Intuition dimension—have very low activity in the fusiform gyrus. As I'll describe in chapter 7, we have discovered why that is and therefore what can be done to change the inputs to the brain in order to raise activity in the fusiform gyrus and thereby nudge someone toward the Socially Intuitive end of the Social Intuition dimension.

When I explain to audiences and classes that people have distinct Emotional Styles and that these styles reflect specific patterns of brain activity, they often assume that Emotional Style must therefore be fixed and, probably, genetically based. Indeed, for decades neuroscientists assumed that the adult brain is essentially fixed in form and function. But we now know that this picture of a static, unchanging brain is wrong. Instead, the brain has a property called neuroplasticity, the ability to change its structure and function in significant ways. That change can come about in response to the experiences we have as well as to the thoughts we think. The brains of virtuoso violinists, for example, show a measurable increase in the size and activity of areas that control the fingers, and the brains of London taxicab drivers, who learn to navigate the insanely complicated network of streets (twenty-five thousand of them!) in that city, show a significant growth in the hippocampus, an area associated with context and spatial memory. Playing the piano and learning a city map are examples of intense, repeated sensory and learning experiences in the outside world.

But the brain can also change in response to messages generated internally—in other words, to our thoughts and intentions. These changes include altering the function of brain regions, expanding or contracting the amount of neural territory devoted to particular tasks, strengthening or weakening connections between different brain regions, increasing or decreasing the level of activity in specific brain circuits, and modulating the neurochemical messenger service that continuously courses through the brain.

My favorite example of how "mere" thought can change the brain in fundamental ways is an experiment I'll call the virtual piano study. Scientists led by Alvaro Pascual-Leone, of Harvard University, had half a group of volunteers learn a simple five-finger keyboard piece, practicing over and over for a week with their right hand. They then used neuroimaging to determine how much of the motor cortex was responsible for moving those fingers, finding that the intense practice had expanded the relevant region. That was not too surprising, since other experiments had found that learning specific movements causes such an expansion. But the scientists had the other half of their group of volunteers only imagine playing the notes; they did not actually touch the ivories. Then the researchers measured whether the motor cortex had noticed. It had. The region that controls the fingers of the right hand had expanded in the virtual pianists just as it had in the volunteers who had actually played the piano. Thinking, and thinking alone, had increased the amount of space the motor cortex devoted to a specific function.

Given that Emotional Style is the product of all these brain functions—connections, circuits, structure/function relationships, and neurochemistry—the implication is undeniable: Since the brain contains the physical underpinnings of Emotional Style, and since the brain can change in these fundamental ways, Emotional Style can change. Yes, our Emotional Style is the result of brain circuitry that is laid down in our early years by the genes we inherited from our parents and by the experiences we have. But that circuitry is not forever fixed. Although Emotional Style is ordinarily quite stable over time, it can be altered by serendipitous experiences as well as by conscious, intentional effort at any point in life, through the intentional cultivation of specific mental qualities or habits.

I am not saying that it is *theoretically* possible to shift your place on one of the continua of Emotional Style, or that such a shift is possible only *in principle*. In my research, I have discovered practical, effective ways to do so. I'll explain more in chapter 11, but for now let it suffice to say that you can modify your Emotional Style to improve your resilience, social intuition, sensitivity to your own internal emotional and physiological states, coping mechanisms, attention, and sense of well-being. The amazing fact is that through mental activity alone we can intentionally change our own brains. Mental activity, ranging from meditation to cognitive-behavior therapy, can alter brain function in specific circuits, with the result that you can develop a broader awareness of social signals, a deeper sensitivity to your own feelings and bodily sensations, and a more consistently positive outlook. In short, through mental training you can alter your patterns of brain activity and the very structure of your brain in a way that will change your Emotional Style and improve your life. I believe this is the ultimate step in mind-body interaction.

You're Perfect: Now Change

There is no ideal Emotional Style, no optimal position on any of the continua that describe the six Emotional Styles, let alone all of them. Civilization couldn't flourish without different emotional types, including the extremes— accountants whose prefrontal cortex and striatum drive them to zip through 1040s while effortlessly blocking distracting messages from the emotional centers of the brain, for instance, and techno geniuses who are more comfortable working with machines than with people because the circuit responsible for social cognition is underactive, making social interactions unimportant to them. Although society labels the accountant "obsessive" and the techie "social-phobic," the world would be a poorer place without them. We need all types.

That said, I am not in the "I'm okay, you're okay" camp that believes every psychological style is equal and equally desirable. You may have noticed in the descriptions of the six dimensions of Emotional Style that some extremes sound almost dysfunctional, such as when a complete lack of Resilience makes someone so slow to recover from adversity that she is at risk for depression. Even when your Emotional Style does not leave you vulnerable to actual mental illness, there is no denying the fact that, at least in twenty-first-century Western culture, some Emotional Styles simply make it harder to be a productive member of society, to forge meaningful relationships, and to achieve a sense of well-being. There may be instances in which being Puzzled rather than Socially Intuitive, Opaque on the Self-Awareness dimension, and Tuned

Out when it comes to Sensitivity to Context is desirable; if nothing else, some of the world's greatest works of art and most monumental achievements in mathematics and science sprang from the tortured minds of social misfits. But with the rare exceptions of the Tolstoys and Hemingways and Van Goghs among us, it is simply harder to lead a meaningful, productive life with some Emotional Styles than with others.

And that, I argue, should be the test. Don't let anyone else tell you that you need to become more Socially Intuitive, for instance, or that you must alter your Attention style from Unfocused to Focused. (Although if your significant other makes the suggestion, you might want to at least give it some thought.) Only if your Emotional Style interferes with your daily life and constrains your happiness, only if it prevents you from reaching your goals or causes you distress, should you consider making an effort to change it. But if you do decide to change, my research has shown that there are specific, effective ways for you to achieve your goal, forms of mental training that can shift patterns of brain activity in a way that can move you closer to where you want to be on the dimensions of Emotional Style.

But we are getting ahead of ourselves. First, it is time to turn to how I first saw the glimmerings of what would become Emotional Style.

CHAPTER 2

■ ■ ■

The Discovery of Emotional Style

To say that studying emotions was not very popular when I began my graduate work in the psychology department at Harvard University in 1972 is like saying the Sahara is a trifle dry. Hardly any scientists would touch the subject. For one thing, the 1970s marked the ascendance of cognitive psychology (a term that had only been coined in 1965). This branch of psychology asks questions about how people perceive, remember, solve problems, speak, and the like, and it was dead serious about the computer as a metaphor for the human mind. Computers do their calculations without emotions, of course, so cognitive psychologists at the time viewed emotions as little more than static that got in the way of the mental processes they wanted to understand.

Some of the most prominent researchers in psychology declared that emotion disrupts cognitive function. The most charitable view of emotion among cognitive psychologists was that emotion is an "interrupt": It occurs when behavior needs to be interrupted so that the organism will pay attention to some key piece of information and alter that behavior. In this view, we feel fear when we see a snake on the path ahead of us because fear causes us to focus on the threat and get the heck out of there. Or we feel sadness when someone we love is hurt because it interrupts whatever we are doing and causes us to attend to his needs. Or we feel anger when someone insults us because anger causes us to focus on this foe and defend ourselves. This view pitted emotion against cognition, casting emotion as a disruptive (albeit occasionally useful) force. Overall, though, there just wasn't much room for emotions in the cold, hard calculus of cognitive psychology, which considered them downright suspect. The attitude was basically one of haughty disdain that this riffraff occupied the same brain that gave rise to cognition. The idea that emotions might be beneficial, or have any function other than interrupting behavior, was antithetical to the idea of emotions as mental distractions and disruptions.

Almost all the research on the brain and emotion at this time was done on lab rats. The studies showed that fear, curiosity, "approach behavior" (in which an animal is attracted to, say, food or a mate, and which is regarded as the closest thing to the human emotion of happiness or desire), and anxiety all reflect activity in the limbic region and the brain stem, particularly the hypothalamus. This small structure sits just above the brain stem and signals the body to generate many of the visceral and hormonal changes that frequently accompany emotion. In a typical study, the experimenter would destroy a certain part of a rat's hypothalamus and observe that the animal no longer showed fear in response to, say, the sight of a cat. Destroying a different part of the hypothalamus left the rat completely uninterested in sex, or feeding, or fighting. All these behaviors were thought to require some kind of drive, or motivation, on an animal's part—hence the inference that the hypothalamus is the font of motivation and, because motivation is considered a part of emotion, perhaps of other emotions, too. (Later, scientists would discover that the hypothalamus is actually not directly involved in generating motivation but is a mere way station for signals originating elsewhere in the brain.)

Since the hypothalamus sits below the cortex, the most recent part of the brain evolutionarily, it was regarded with some scorn. I call it cortical snobbism: If a function arose from activity in any region other than the exalted cortex, it must be primitive and somehow antithetical to cognition. This sort of thinking spurred a great debate in psychology that reached its apex in the 1980s, pitting cognition against emotion and viewing them as separate and antagonistic systems of the mind and brain.

In addition to the belief that emotions play no role in the thinking machine that is the human mind, the other obstacle to studying emotions back then was that psychology was just emerging from the long, dark night that saw the hegemony of behaviorism, the school that emphasizes only external behavior and is content to ignore everything else. Emotional *behavior* is fair game to behaviorists, but because emotions themselves are internal, they are suspect, deemed unfit for the polite company of "real" psychological phenomena. As a result, the only significant research on human emotions centered on observations that Charles Darwin had made in the mid-nineteenth century. Although best known for his discovery of natural selection as the driving force of evolution, Darwin also dabbled in human and animal emotion, studying in particular the facial expressions that reflect what someone is feeling. In the 1970s, a handful of psychologists continued in this tradition, by parsing facial expressions into the tiniest components possible—individual muscles that produce a frown or a smile or other expression. Facial expressions were at least an observable behavior and thus fair game in the behaviorist paradigm. Significantly, however, the work on facial expressions made no reference to the brain . . . whose mysterious workings were dismissed by behaviorism as off-limits to rigorous empirical research.

Sweet Dreams

Yet even in the 1970s I had seen that hidden, internal phenomena can be coaxed out into the daylight. During my senior year in high school, in Brooklyn, I volunteered at a sleep laboratory at nearby Maimonides Medical Center, which happened to be the hospital where I was born. Study participants would show up in the evening, and after one of the scientists in charge explained that they were to sleep normally—or as close to normally as one can in a strange room on a strange bed with strangers going in and out and a Medusa's head of wires pasted to your scalp—they would retreat to a private room. Chuck, one of the researchers, would paste electrodes all over the volunteer's face and scalp. Electrodes on the scalp monitor brain waves. Electrodes around the eyes detect the rapid eye movements that occur during dreaming. Electrodes elsewhere on the face measure muscle activity (just watch your sleeping companion some night and you'll see that muscles of the cheeks, lips, and forehead dance with activity during some phases of sleep). Chuck would make sure the electronics were working, wish the subject sweet dreams, and start the "polygraph," a hulking machine whose thirty-two pens recorded all the physiological measures on a continuous stream of paper that moved along at about an inch every second. That's where I hung out. My august job was to ensure that the pens were filled with ink and properly flowing. Let me say in my own defense that this was not as easy as it might sound: The pens frequently clogged, which required inserting a thin wire into the eye of the pen to clean it out. My introduction to scientific methodology.

Usually the participants were asleep within minutes, and EEG—electroencephalogram, or brain wave—data began streaming into the control room. I loved seeing the squiggly line EEG traces indicating that the person had fallen into rapid eye movement (REM) sleep. Once I mastered the whole pen-maintenance thing, I was rewarded with the job of waking the sleeping person, by calling his name over the intercom, and asking what had been going on in his mind just before he was awakened. I was intrigued by the connection between the spikes and squiggles of the EEG and the fantastic images and bizarre narratives of the dreams. Though I can't recall any of the details of the dreams, I do remember very vividly being impressed that virtually every dream contained significant emotion—terror or joy, anger, sadness, jealousy, or hatred. This experience in the sleep lab also showed me that one successful path to understanding the mind was studying the brain. Even to the fifteen-year-old me, the message was clear: Purely internal mental processes (brain waves and the emotional component of dreams) with no external manifestations are demonstrably real and can be studied in the laboratory. Contrary to the behaviorists' claims, you didn't need behavior—in the sense of an action observable by a third party—to have a valid psychological phenomenon.

This suspicion grew stronger during my years as an undergraduate at New York University, where I was double majoring in psychology and a small interdisciplinary program called the Metropolitan Leadership Program, which emphasized small seminars rather than big lecture courses. It was during these years that my youthful conviction that psychology needed to study and explain internal mental processes in order to be a true science of the mind ran smack into the wall of Authority.

The chairman of the NYU Department of Psychology at the time was Charles Catania, a dyed-in-the-wool behaviorist. Catania taught an honors seminar that I took, and after class he and I would often get into tussles about the fundamental nature of psychology. Catania argued that only behaviors observable by a third party constitute scientific data and thus a proper subject of study for psychology. I, however, cockily insisted that what the behaviorists were studying is a very small sliver of psychological reality. What about what people *felt*, I asked? How could that be ignored? And what about this textbook I was reading for an abnormal psychology course, which (in true behaviorist fashion) smugly declared psychiatric disorders to be the consequences of screwy reinforcement contingencies? In other words, it blamed serious mental illnesses such as depression, bipolar disorder, and schizophrenia on aberrant rewards and punishments, asserting that people who hear voices or ride an uncontrolled emotional roller coaster or feel such black despair that they contemplate suicide are doing so because they have been rewarded for it or were punished for being "normal." That argument is not only morally abhorrent, I argued to Catania, but it ignores biology and, specifically, the brain! I certainly didn't convert Catania from behaviorism (though I did drop the abnormal psych course after a week). But the back-and-forth helped sharpen my own focus and convinced me that something more profound than overt behavior was waiting for psychological research to discover.

What science had discovered so far about the inner life of the mind was, shall we say, underwhelming, as I learned while doing research for an undergraduate paper on personality. This was my first exposure to the existing scientific literature on emotion. Most of the human studies were being conducted by social psychologists who held that emotion comprises dual fundamental constituents. The first is physiological arousal—things like how fast your heart beats when you are afraid or how red your face gets when you feel angry. Physiological arousal supposedly provides the energetic, or oomph, component of the emotion—whether you are mildly annoyed or grab-a-gun furious, slightly envious or murderously jealous. The second ingredient of emotion in this early scheme is cognitive appraisal. As the name implies, this is the process of observing the aforementioned racing heart or red face and thinking to yourself, *Aha, I guess I feel afraid* (or angry). The idea was that physiological arousal is nonspecific and undifferentiated; being happy *feels* the same as being angry or surprised or scared or filled with jealousy. Only the cognitive interpretation of that arousal tells you what the heck you are feeling.

Put this way—and I am exaggerating only a little—you can see how ridiculous this model is. The idea that there is fundamentally no qualitative physiological difference among emotions, that there is no difference in how it *feels* to be happy or angry or sad or jealous, and that what distinguishes one emotion from another is solely the cognitive interpretations or thoughts people have about their internal arousal, seemed wrong to me, both personally and scientifically. I was dissatisfied enough with this model to investigate whether psychologists had always thought this way. I began reading William James's chapter on emotion in his seminal two-volume tome of 1890, *The Principles of Psychology.* James proposes that emotion is the perception of bodily change. In his model, fear, for example, primarily comes from the perception that our hearts are beating faster and/or that we are frozen in place, unable to move. The internal bodily changes are provoked by the environment—in this example, a shadowy figure in a doorway up ahead—and the emotion consists of the perception of these bodily changes. For James, then, different emotions have *different* physiological signatures; they could not be simply the undifferentiated physiological arousal that the prevailing model claimed.

Another inspiration for my budding interest in the science of emotion was the thrill I felt when I discovered that Darwin wrote an entire book about emotion in 1872, *The Expression of the Emotions in Man and Animals* (you can now download it free, since it is in the public domain). By emphasizing the distinctive signs of emotion, particularly facial expressions, Darwin reinforced my tentative ideas that different emotions must be associated with distinct physiological profiles. After I read Darwin, I was convinced of three things: that emotion is central to understanding the important qualities of being human, that the dominant approach to emotion in human psychology was seriously flawed, and that the brain somehow had to be the focus of any study of emotion. A complete understanding of the mind, I believed, was simply impossible without a complete understanding of emotion. If science couldn't figure out emotion, it would never figure out personality, temperament, illnesses such as anxiety disorders and depression, or (possibly) cognition. I was equally sure that the key to the wonderful mysteries of human emotion lay in the brain.

Despite my heresy, NYU awarded me a degree in psychology. I set my sights on graduate school, but my iconoclasm and, in particular, my insistence on bringing the brain into the study of emotion did not make it easy to find the right fit. I was attracted to Stanford University and went out to visit. There I met psychology professor Ernest "Jack" Hilgard, a famous and fascinating character (he had matriculated at Yale Divinity School before switching to the psychology department) who had made his mark with contributions to the theory of learning—and, later, to hypnosis, especially how it can be used to control pain. I was intrigued by the idea of studying with Hilgard, but he discouraged me from going to Stanford: There was really no one in the psychology department who was doing any biological research in humans, he warned me. I did apply to the Graduate Center of the City University of New York, where I think I would have been quite content, but I also applied to Harvard.

During the interview process there, I had a wonderful discussion with Gary Schwartz, who was studying psychophysiology. Now we were getting closer to the brain: The "physiology" in that discipline referred to bodily changes such as heart rate and blood pressure. I also had an interview with psychology professor David McClelland, who was well known around campus for his involvement in the Ram Dass affair a decade earlier. David had been the director of the Center for Research in Personality, which supported research by a young faculty member named Richard Alpert—research that involved giving psychedelic drugs such as psilocybin to undergraduates. (Timothy Leary, of LSD fame, was Alpert's coinvestigator in the research.) Harvard eventually took a dim view of this study, especially since Alpert frequently took the drug himself, which critics suggested might make it difficult for him to accurately observe its effects on his volunteers, and since a couple of students in the study landed in a mental hospital. In 1963 the university fired Alpert, who eventually changed his name to Ram Dass.

I was faintly aware of all this, which piqued my curiosity about McClelland even more and emboldened me to bring up a topic that, if broached with any other eminent psychology researcher, might have sunk my chances at admission. I had recently read Carl Jung's autobiography, *Memories, Dreams, Reflections*, which made a big impression on me. I knew that mainstream psychology had pretty much shunned Jung because of his unconventional ideas on, for instance, the collective unconscious and the theory of archetypes, yet I found some of his observations very insightful, particularly those about individual differences. Jung was really the first psychologist to discuss introversion and extraversion as traits and to speculate about psychological and physiological differences among people of each type. Somehow in my conversation with McClelland we ended up discussing Jung. I was so impressed that this renowned Harvard psychology professor was open to such ideas, it reinforced my intuition that Harvard was the right place for me. So off I went, determined to plunge into research on the brain and emotions. I was not going to let the prospect of working in an academic backwater (the topic, not Harvard) deter me.

On to Harvard

When I showed up for graduate school and told my adviser, Gary Schwartz, that I hoped to study the brain basis of emotion, he was skeptical. Like most psychology researchers at the time, Gary didn't know much about brain physiology. (He had never done an EEG, which measures basic brain electrical activity, until I arrived.) I found it bizarre that mainstream psychological research—and Harvard epitomized the mainstream, which at that time meant behaviorism—had so little interest in how the brain generates emotion. After all, unless someone discovers how, say, the appendix produces and processes emotions, the brain is *it* when it comes to organs of emotion. Yet the precious little psychological research on emotion back then was based on the study of facial expressions (classic behaviorism!) or answers from questionnaires, neither of which I thought would ever get us to the essence of emotion. Incredibly, the brain was never mentioned in these studies. The lack of interest on the part of academic scientists in the role and function of the brain in emotions was as weird to me as if I had stumbled into a department of nephrology and found they had no interest in kidneys. Even weirder was that William James, considered the founder of the science of psychology (and, ironically, the namesake of the fifteen-story building that houses Harvard's psych department), explains in the preface to *The Principles of Psychology* that the brain is the one bodily organ underlying all mental operations. He then makes the profound assertion that the rest of *Principles*—all 1,328 pages—is but a footnote to this claim. Harvard's psychology researchers apparently hadn't gotten the memo.

I got a firsthand view of the behaviorist paradigm that had the Harvard psych department in a death grip one day when, during my first week as a grad student, I stepped into an elevator in William James Hall. There stood B. F. Skinner, the founding father of behaviorism, with his six-foot-plus frame and trademark shaggy white hair. Flustered, I pressed the button for my floor and immediately realized I'd made a mistake. Mumbling, "I changed my mind," I pressed a different floor. To which Skinner said, "Son, you didn't change your mind; you changed your behavior."

There was, however, a silver lining in psychology's lack of interest in the brain basis of emotion. When I arrived for graduate work intent on studying the role of the brain in people's emotional lives, the amount of scientific literature on the topic was, shall we say, not exactly intimidating. Unlike the many grad students who struggle to come up with an original topic for their thesis research (with no disrespect to English lit scholars, is there anything original—and important—left to say about *King Lear*?), I wasn't going to have that problem. I had the rare opportunity to define my own field of study, and it would be all but impossible for some authority to criticize me for failing to adhere to the prevailing paradigm; there *was* no prevailing paradigm for the neural bases of emotion. The challenge was the opposite: what to pick from the plethora of unanswered—really, unstudied—questions about how emotions work.

There were two wells I could draw from. The first was research in animals. In these studies, scientists selectively destroyed or stimulated (with implanted electrodes) certain brain regions to see which areas are correlated with which emotions (or what passes for emotion in animals: we think we know when an animal is expressing fear, rage, or contentment and assume the animal is feeling the emotion at least somewhat the way humans do). Most of these studies, going back to the nineteenth century, focused on the role of the hypothalamus, as I mentioned above.

The second source of knowledge about emotions came from the study of patients who had suffered damage to a specific, localized region of the brain, with the result that their emotional life had been knocked for a loop. Perhaps the best-known example was Phineas Gage. A railroad foreman, Gage was overseeing a crew working on the Rutland and Burlington Railroad near Cavendish, Vermont, in 1848. To clear the track bed in order to lay rail, the crew drilled holes into the large boulders they needed to remove, filled them with dynamite, inserted a fuse, and used a tamping iron to plug the hole with sand so that the force of the blast would be directed into the rock. Unfortunately, while Gage was tamping down sand with the iron, a spark ignited the dynamite. The resulting explosion shot the thirteen-pound, forty-four-inch-long tamping iron straight into Gage's skull under the left cheekbone. It went through his brain, exiting through the top of his head and landing thirty yards away.

Although the bar impaled his frontal lobes, Gage not only survived but, after convulsing for a minute, sat up and asked his men for the logbook he used to keep records of his crew's hours. He was even able to walk to an oxcart that took him to his boardinghouse; there, a local physician tended to his wounds, removing shards of bone and replacing skull fragments that had been blown off by the tamping iron. Gage seemed to recover, but his survival quickly took a dark turn. His wife and friends began noticing that their soft-spoken, reliable, modest, even-keeled Phineas had become erratic, fitful, and prone to unprovoked and profanity-filled rages, "pertinaciously obstinate, yet capricious and vacillating," his doctor wrote. Once "the most efficient and capable foreman," Gage had become "impatient of restraint of advice when it conflicts with his desires, . . . devising many plans of future operation, which are no sooner arranged than they are abandoned. . . . [H]is friends and acquaintances said he was 'no longer Gage.'" The reason eventually became clear: The prefrontal region of the brain impaled by the bar is the locus of emotional control and similar high-order cognitive function. Phineas Gage's brain gave neuroscientists their first evidence that specific brain structures control specific mental functions and suggested a key role for the prefrontal cortex in the regulation of emotions.

While the findings from animal research and studies of brain-damaged humans were interesting and important, they did not bear directly on the brain mechanisms implicated in *normal* emotion in humans.

Inspiration Strikes

The 1970s were the days when scientists spent a lot of time in the library since research journals existed only as printed volumes, not as electron patterns in a box on your desk (or a Flash Gordon–type gadget that fit in your pocket). I spent many nights every week in Harvard Medical School's Countway Library, which is in Boston across the Charles River from Harvard's main campus in Cambridge. I was there so much I had my own carrel, and I loved browsing journals and xeroxing articles—hundreds and hundreds of them—as I devoured the scientific literature. One of the best parts was the serendipity factor, stumbling onto journals that I would never have intentionally searched through but that were in plain sight on the shelves, beckoning me to take a look: *The Anatomical Record, American Journal of Physical Anthropology, Radiology.* . . . I would go into the stacks and look through journals and books a hundred years old, their musty smell transporting me back to the science of another era.

It was on one of my nocturnal perambulations through Countway's basement stacks, during my first year in graduate school, that I happened to pull down the August 1972 issue of the journal *Cortex*. In it I found a paper by an Italian neurologist at the University of Perugia named Guido Gainotti. He studied patients who had sustained localized damage to either the right or left hemisphere of their brain, looking in particular at how that damage affected their emotions. What he found was "pathological laughter and crying"—"pathological" meaning inappropriate, since the patients were not responding to what the rest of us would call funny (such as a great joke) or heartbreaking (being dumped by a lover). Instead, they would burst into laughter or tears at completely random and often inappropriate moments. What Gainotti found was that patients who had sustained damage to the left side of the brain in the front (mostly because of stroke) exhibited pathological crying, as well as some of the symptoms we see in patients with depression, such as a lack of drive and an inability to set goals and persevere in reaching them. In contrast, patients whose brain injury occurred in the right frontal region exhibited pathological laughter.

This study captivated me because it held out the tantalizing possibility that particular brain regions and brain networks could be shown to generate specific emotions. As soon as I read it I felt I'd found the secret passage to an enchanted kingdom. I began to wonder: If damage to the left frontal region produces pathological crying and symptoms of depression, then is the left frontal region responsible for some emotional quality (such as optimism or resilience) that is lacking in depression? That wasn't the obvious implication it might seem like today, when we're used to linking brain functions to emotional and other mental states. In fact, Gainotti interpreted his finding differently. He thought that damage to the right hemisphere was somehow interfering with a patient's understanding of his neurological condition, and this was producing inappropriately positive emotion in the face of severe neurological injury. But the brash first-year graduate student that I was didn't think the scientist who discovered this phenomenon—that damage to particular brain areas produces location-specific emotional change—was owed any particular deference when it came to grasping the implications of his own finding. I focused on the possibility that the left prefrontal region might be the seat of positive emotion, and that damaging it leads to a depressive state.

Left, Right, Left, Right

I wish I could say that this insight inspired me then and there to map out a plan of experimental research on the brain basis of human emotion, but it didn't. I did, however, get my feet wet, so to speak. With Gary's blessing, I ran an experiment that combined, in a very primitive way, the ideas of laterality and emotion that Gainotti had touched on. One of the few observations psychologists had about laterality was that when a person is asked a question that requires some reflection, the direction the eyes move indicates which of the brain's two hemispheres is working on the answer. If the left brain is working on the answer while the right brain lazes around (as usually happens if the answer has to do with verbal ability), the eyes tend to move to the right. If the right brain gets the call (as it typically does if the answer requires spatial reasoning), then the eyes move to the left. (Definitely try this at home. Just be sure the question can't be answered automatically but requires some thought. I've gotten good results with "Think of three synonyms for stubborn" and "How many corners does a cube have?")

In this rudimentary experiment, I asked participants a series of questions, some meant to trigger an emotion ("When was the last time you were angry?") and some neutral ("What did you have for breakfast this morning?"). As they answered, I recorded in which direction their eyes moved. When participants were presented with emotional questions, I found, they looked more to the left—indicative of right hemisphere activation—compared with responses to neutral questions. By chance, however, my test included more negative than positive emotional questions, so when I say that participants looked to the left in response to emotional questions, I should actually say that they looked to the left in response to emotionally *negative* questions. I had thus stumbled upon one of our first clues that the right hemisphere might be more activated during negative than positive emotion. With Gary and a Harvard undergraduate named Foster Maer, I published the paper in the prestigious journal *Science*.

Once this study was completed it was clear I needed better, more precise measures of localized brain activity. Eye movements might provide a crude index of which hemisphere is more activated, but it provides no information on which regions within a hemisphere are involved. Getting better measurements was a challenge. In the 1970s few scientific tools were available to probe the human brain noninvasively—that is, without opening up the skull and sticking things into the brain. Wilder Penfield had famously done it that way, mapping the brains of patients undergoing surgery for epilepsy by removing part of the skull to reveal the brain and then applying tiny jolts of electricity to different spots to see what the patient would feel or do. With one zap, a patient would recall a vivid memory of a visiting nephew who was putting on his hat and coat to go home; zapping another region would cause the patient to feel as if her right forearm had been touched, or would cause an arm or leg or finger to move unbidden, as if the patient were a marionette. (I'll have more to say about Penfield's brain mapping in chapter 8.) One of his most interesting observations was that when he stimulated the anterior temporal lobe, an area of the cortex that lies near the amygdala, patients often reported feeling emotions.

Since I had no plans to become a brain surgeon, however, probing the cortex for sites relevant to emotions was not exactly an option for me. I needed a less invasive method for observing what was going on in the brain. The period

of the 1970s was decades before the advent of neuroimaging technology—
devices such as PET and fMRI—that produces the multicolored brain scans
that so enchant the public (and neuroscientists). My only option was therefore
to measure the electrical signals from the brain using sensors on the scalp, the
technique used to record EEGs.

You might think that the electrical signals zipping around the brain would
have no more chance of being detected on the outside of the skull than the
whispers of two robbers in a bank vault would have of being heard by a guard
patrolling the other side. In fact, however, external electrodes can act as antennae and do pick up the brain's electrical chitchat. And you don't have to remove any slabs of skull to do it. Another advantage of pasting electrodes to
the skull is that they give you excellent time resolution. By that, I mean that
even if an electrical signal in the brain lasts only a tiny fraction of a second (to
be precise, as little as fifty milliseconds, or thousandths of a second), the electrode will detect it. Since I thought the emotions I was planning to induce in
my volunteers might be pretty fleeting, good time resolution would be critical.

Unfortunately, much as the Heisenberg uncertainty principle says that if
you want to measure a particle's location precisely, you have to settle for not
knowing its speed; in the case of neuroimaging, if you want to know precisely
when a fleeting moment of brain activity occurred, then you have to settle for
imprecision in *where* it occurred. (And if you want to know precisely *where*
activity occurred, you have to accept not knowing precisely *when* it occurred.)
So while I could know within milliseconds when my volunteers experienced
an emotion, I could know only within centimeters where in the brain the neurons generated that emotion. Centimeters can mean the difference between the
temporal lobe and the frontal lobe. (In fact, calculating even roughly where the
electrical activity originated requires sophisticated mathematical techniques,
which fortunately were being developed by physicists around the same time I
was hunting for new measurement methods.)

Gary Schwartz's lab had never previously used measures of brain electrical
activity in research, so we had to lay a lot of groundwork to demonstrate that
we could rely on EEGs to determine the source of specific brain activity. We
presented simple visual and kinesthetic stimuli—flashing lights and tapping
on the forearm—to twenty participants and then asked them to imagine those
stimuli. All the while we recorded brain electrical activity through electrodes

on the scalp. Thank God our electrodes picked up activity in the visual cortex when the participants imagined the flashing light, and activity in the somatosensory cortex when they imagined the tapping. Anything else and it would have been back to the drawing board.

Now we were ready to sic EEG on emotion. But how? I proposed to Gary that we have undergraduates (always in abundant supply on a college campus) call up two kinds of emotional memories—relaxing and angry—while we recorded their EEG and heart rate. The heart rate measurement would tell us if they were lying about which memory they had called up, we figured, since heart rate is higher when people remember a knock-down, drag-out argument with their father than when they recall seeing the baby ducks in Boston's Public Garden. Again, the science gods smiled on us: We could indeed differentiate between a positive and negative emotion using measures of brain electrical activity as recorded by an EEG. This was the first published study in which EEGs had detected people's interior emotional states.

I now had several substantial publications under my belt, including one on the direction of eye gaze and emotion, and numerous articles on EEG changes during emotion and cognition—but the world wasn't very impressed. As I neared the end of graduate school, I had few job offers. My interdisciplinary interests were simply too broad for most psychology departments, and I did not fit the then-prevailing molds of either behaviorism or cognitive psych. Everyone was perfectly polite and interested in my work—or so they said— but they eventually told me that it was too physiological for their cognitive psychology program or too cognitive for their physiological psychology program. (I felt no small measure of vindication when, in 1995, Harvard tried to recruit me back as a full professor. It was a very attractive offer, but for a variety of reasons I politely declined.) Fortunately, however, I received an offer from the State University of New York at Purchase, a town in suburban Westchester County about twenty-five miles north of Manhattan. This then-new campus of the SUNY system promised to be an interdisciplinary haven. I accepted.

Excedrin Headache Number One

The Natural Science Building on the Purchase campus had just been completed, and with the new facility came a cornucopia of electronics—logic gates and oscillators and other goodies just begging to be hooked up into a state-of-the-art electrophysiology lab. Since I had my hands full with all the responsibilities of a new assistant professor, I needed someone to build me a lab. Let me introduce you to Cliff Saron.

Cliff was a sophomore biology major at Harvard when I was a graduate student there. We met in 1973 at a conference of the Association for Humanistic Psychology in Quebec, and the following semester Cliff took Gary Schwartz's course on psychophysiology, which included instruction on how to measure brain function with EEGs. Cliff was very interested in altered states of consciousness and in how biology gives rise to consciousness, but it was his facility with electronics that really made him stand out. He had been a bit of a phone phreaker as a teenager in New York City (the 1970s version of a computer hacker; Cliff learned that if you play a whistle of a specific frequency [2600 hertz, for those who want to try this at home] into a phone receiver, you can disconnect one call and connect to someone else) and worked in theater sound and radio engineering in high school and college. This put him in the perfect position to take the lead in setting up the equipment we needed to do electrophysiology, recording electrical activity in the brain.

Cliff also took a class on the psychology of consciousness, which my friend Daniel Goleman and I taught. That course was notable for many things, but what truly stood out was that in one of the class's discussion sections the students and instructors meditated. (I'll have more to say about the roots of my interest in meditation and consciousness in chapter 9.) Dan would go on to have a stellar career at the *New York Times* covering psychology and to write the mega-selling book *Emotional Intelligence*. Cliff graduated from Harvard College around the same time that I got my Ph.D. and headed off to Purchase.

As luck would have it, Dan, who was then working as an editor at the magazine *Psychology Today*, took pity on me for my paucity of job offers and my inability to get research grants through normal channels. He managed to persuade the advertising agency that had the Bristol-Myers Squibb account to give me a grant to evaluate Excedrin commercials. What the company wanted was to see if the current modern methods of recording brain activity could provide useful information about the effectiveness of their television spots. For instance, if brain circuitry associated with disgust became active while someone watched the commercial, that would be a bad thing; circuitry associated with desire, good. (The ad agency was far ahead of its time: Measuring brain responses to ads has taken off in the new century and is now called neuromarketing.)

With the $75,000 grant, a significant amount of money back then, I was able to hire Cliff to build my lab, using the goodies that the new Natural Science Building came with as well as a signal averager (a device for measuring small changes in brain electrical activity evoked by external stimuli, such as sights and sounds) that a friend at Harvard Medical School had given me as a sort of going-away present. Cliff and I flew from Boston to New York with this thing as carry-on luggage. It was as big as a moderate-size television set and had enough dials and lights and cables that if I tried to carry it onto a plane these days, I would be hauled off for questioning. As we built the lab, it was like "The Hardy Boys Do Electrophysiology." (I was the Hardy Boy who needed to be kept away from dangerous equipment: I had accidentally set fire to my lab in William James Hall one day during an experiment. Although no one was hurt, some equipment was torched, and I had no desire to repeat the experience.)

The ad agency basically told me, "If you evaluate our commercials, you can have the TV programs that come between them and do whatever you want with them." (Most of us think of commercials as interrupting TV programs, but advertisers seem to view programs as interrupting their commercials.) While we of course did the research the company paid for, we were much more interested in the impact of the emotional content of the programming. The tape included episodes of *The Carol Burnett Show* and news footage about a mining accident complete with anxious wives and children racing from their homes to the town square when a siren signaled an underground disaster. In other words, our funders supplied us with video clips that were perfect for inducing a good mood, in the first case, and anxiety and fear in the second case. This provided a great opportunity to determine if brain electrical signals, recorded from the scalp, could differentiate between positive and negative emotions.

Cliff fitted the volunteers with sensors on the muscles of the forehead and around the eyes (the muscles that produce a frown or a squint), as well as a cap containing sixteen electrodes. Then we got them comfortably situated in front of a television on which we played the Carol Burnett and lost-miner clips; the first would reliably induce a positive emotion such as contentment or amusement, and the second would reliably induce a negative emotion such as fear or anger. By "reliably," I mean that I had pretested the clips on other volunteers, asking them what emotion each clip induced. If a clip made some people angry and others amused, for instance, or if the induced emotion was weak ("Well, maybe I was a little worried about the miners, but not really"), it didn't make the cut. Only unambiguously and strongly positive- or negative-emotion-inducing clips were included in the experiment.

While the participants viewed the videos, we monitored the brain electrical signals that the electrodes in the skullcap were picking up to make sure everything was working. The EEG output went to electronic filters and then to a Rube Goldberg device that, every thirty seconds or so, spewed out numbers indicating the average amount of energy in the brain waves we were interested in. (The greater the energy, or amplitude, of the wave, the more intense the brain activity.) We then hand-entered these numbers onto punch cards and fed them into a computer that filled half the room. Cliff had also rigged up a button for the volunteers to press—hard if they felt an emotion strongly, and softly if they felt the emotion weakly. This, in addition to the facial movements, allowed us to focus on brain activity that accompanied clear and powerful conscious emotional reactions.

We found that when volunteers viewed clips previously rated as inducing positive emotion and moved their smile muscles, regions in the left prefrontal cortex became highly activated. Watching clips rated as inducing strong negative emotions while showing expressions of fear or disgust activated the right prefrontal region. I was relieved to see that our findings jibed perfectly with those of Gainotti, who had reported that injury to the left side of the brain induced pathological crying, and injury to the right side induced pathological laughter. If people cry for no apparent reason because the part of their brain that sustains positive emotions has been knocked out, then his work points to the left side of the brain as the source of positive emotions—just as we found in the volunteers, whose left prefrontal regions went wild for Carol Burnett. Similarly, if people with damage to the right side of the brain succumb to pathological laughter because the right side sustains negative emotions such as fear and disgust, then Gainotti's work points to the right hemisphere as the source of these negative emotions—again as in our volunteers, whose right prefrontal regions were afraid for the miners.

Our findings from this experiment were the first to show that positive and negative emotions are distinguished by activation in the left and right prefrontal cortex, respectively. But to tell you the truth, I didn't quite appreciate what we had. Although I submitted a short version of the results as an abstract to a scientific conference, I never wrote them up for an actual paper. In part, I held back because I felt I didn't have a rigorous way to independently measure the emotion participants were experiencing. That is, we sort of assumed that people found Carol Burnett funny and feared for the miners, but for all we knew some of the volunteers couldn't stand her and others were immune to the miners' plight. Okay, I'm exaggerating—I had no reason to think any of the responses would be that aberrant—but I still felt the experiment lacked the rigor needed for a scientific paper.

Tale of the Tape

So I redid this experiment with much more refined measures of emotion. In what would prove a seminal study, volunteers showed up at my laboratory at SUNY Purchase, where I explained that this was a study of the brain and emotion and that we would be showing them short film clips while we measured their brain electrical activity. I fitted each participant with a cap containing sixteen electrodes (we now use 256) and sat them in front of a television. We then played four two- to three-minute video clips—two that had been shown to induce positive emotions such as amusement or happiness (we used puppies playing with flowers and gorillas in a zoo taking a bath), and two that had been shown to trigger negative emotions such as disgust or fear (we used films from nursing school showing a leg amputation and a third-degree-burn victim). While the participants viewed the videos, I monitored the signals that the electrodes in the skullcap were picking up from their brains.

Unbeknownst to the participants, there was a hidden video camera mounted behind what looked like a loudspeaker. This is where one of my most important collaborators came in. Paul Ekman was a psychologist at the University of California, San Francisco, and probably the leading scientist of emotion at that time. Paul is among the small group of mentors and colleagues who have most influenced my professional development. I first met him in 1974 when, as a graduate student, I was scheduled to give a brief talk at the annual meeting of the International Neuropsychological Society in San Francisco. Over the previous two years, I had read a lot of Paul's seminal studies, which demonstrated that the facial expressions for several basic emotions are human universals. That is, people in cultures as different as New Guinea and Borneo, Japan and Brazil (all of which Paul had traveled to) and the United States, formed the same facial expressions when they felt any of six basic emotions: happiness, sadness, anger, fear, disgust, and surprise. (It is just a coincidence that there are also six dimensions of Emotional Style.) As a result, a native of New Guinea can recognize a disgusted expression on the face of a Parisian, a Peruvian can recognize happiness on the face of an Inuit, and a member of the !Kung San can recognize fear or surprise or sadness or anger on the face of a Tokyoite.

From these discoveries, Paul (who, appropriately, is one of the most emotionally expressive people I know) developed a very detailed system for coding the muscle movements that constitute facial signs of emotion. It is based on the measurement of forty-four independent movements, whose various combinations uniquely describe every facial expression that Homo sapiens are capable of. To develop the system, Paul taught himself to move each of these muscles independently. (Not only is Paul a wonderful scientist, but he is also probably the best facial athlete in the world!) The system has been used by security forces, law enforcement agencies, and others who need to read people's emotions from their faces, often in matters of life or death. Paul's work exploded into pop culture with the January 2009 debut of the Fox television show *Lie to Me*, which was inspired by his research and for which Paul served as a consultant.

During our meeting in San Francisco, Paul and I spent hours talking about emotion, prospects for studying it with neuroscience, and the general state of psychology, and in the early 1980s we began to collaborate, starting with the gorillas/amputation study. We videotaped each participant with the hidden camera, focusing on the face, and recorded brain electrical activity using EEG sensors on the scalp. Paul coded the facial behavior of the participants, recording precisely when different facial signs of emotion first appeared and when they faded. These expressions indicated when a volunteer was experiencing peak emotions. We then determined from the time stamps on the EEG readout which brain electrical signals coincided with each instance of facial behavior. In this way, we began to develop an understanding of the neural correlates of happiness, fear, and disgust—the primary emotions evoked by these clips.

Things got off to a bad start. One of the first things we looked at, since the puppies and gorillas triggered smiles so reliably, was the electrical activity that accompanied all those grins. To my consternation, electrical activity in the brain during the several seconds of a smile was not all that different from brain activity at baseline, when participants were watching nothing more emotionally provocative than a test pattern. How could the brain activity that accompanied happiness, amusement, joy, or whatever else the smiling video watchers were feeling be indistinguishable from the brain activity that accompanied *nothing*? I initially thought that maybe the method of recording brain activity from the scalp was too crude. Or perhaps the cynical senior scientists who were skeptical of this entire approach were right; maybe it was a pipe dream to think I could peer into the brain's emotional machinery by sticking electrodes to people's scalps.

Then I remembered some classical research by the nineteenth-century French anatomist Guillaume Benjamin Armand Duchenne de Boulogne. Duchenne observed that in a smile of true happiness the eye muscles, not just the mouth and cheek muscles, move. That produces a kind of crinkling on the corners of the eyes. (Next time you are chatting with someone, pay particular attention to those spots. If they don't crinkle when the person smiles, it's not a real smile of joy but a social smile. The crinkles mean the person is truly happy, joyful, or amused, and not faking it. Or as Duchenne put it in his 1862 masterpiece *Mécanisme de la physionomie humaine*, "The muscle around the eye does not obey the will; it is only brought into play by a true feeling.")

Paul had been coding smiles solely on the basis of changes in the cheek (zygomatic) muscles that pull the corners of the lips toward the ears. The brain activity that accompanied these movements was a mess. In some participants there were spikes of activity in the left prefrontal region during genuine, cheek-raising smiles, but in other smiling participants no discernible pattern emerged.

As Duchenne discovered, however, it is the eyes and not the cheeks or mouth that convey the true signs of joy. So back we went to the videotape. This time Paul coded smiles based on the eye muscles as well as the zygomatic muscles, a combination producing what we subsequently labeled a "Duchenne smile." Bingo: The data started behaving and making sense. As we compared facial expressions to EEG activity, we saw that when volunteers produced a Duchenne smile they simultaneously showed a pattern of greater left (compared with right) prefrontal activation than they did when they formed both non-Duchenne smiles and no facial expression at all—the baseline state. In a follow-up study, we instructed participants to smile (rather than relying on film clips to make them do so) using either the cheek muscles alone or both the cheek and the eye muscles. Only when both muscle groups participated did we see a shift toward greater left-side activation in the brain. This finding supports the folk wisdom that if you intentionally produce a genuine smile, you will feel happier. We now had brain data to prove it.

I distinctly remember the excitement I felt when I saw the brain correlates of positive and negative emotions. The fact that the activity occurred not in the brain stem and limbic system—primitive regions that have no role in cognition—but in the exalted prefrontal cortex gave me an inkling that we were going to make waves in the scientific community. In its limited thinking about the brain and emotions, psychology had concluded that the hypothalamus and other parts of the limbic system play the starring role (remember those experiments that obliterated a rat's hypothalamus and thus disrupted the animal's emotions). Yet we had fingered the prefrontal cortex. This region was considered the seat of human reason, the locus of forethought and wisdom and rationality and other cognitive functions that distinguish us from "lower" animals. But we were saying it rules our emotions, too—and that the barricade that psychology had erected between reason and emotion has no basis in fact.

From the Brains of Babes

I immediately started to wonder whether this laterality, in which the right prefrontal region supports negative emotions and the left supports positive emotions, develops over many years or is present from the start of life. To find out meant studying babies as young as we could get to sit still. As luck would have it, during a visit to Harvard in 1978 I ran into a former grad-school classmate, Nathan Fox. Nathan had done his graduate work with Jerome Kagan, one of the world's leading developmental psychologists, and had recently moved to New York City to work at Roosevelt Hospital. After chatting for a while in Harvard Yard, we agreed to talk again when we returned to New York. Nathan was interested in childhood temperament and the development of emotion but had never conducted neurological research and did not use any kind of brain measures. I had never studied infants or children. A collaboration was born.

We recruited thirty-eight ten-month-old infants, an age by which babies can clearly recognize faces, by advertising in New York newspapers for a study on the "psychophysiology of emotional development." I didn't trust the film clips we'd been using to induce the emotions we wanted in infants (it takes a more developed comic sensibility to find bathing gorillas amusing, after all), so I decided to go with the basics: video clips of an actress laughing or crying. As in my original study looking for laterality in emotions, I fitted each baby with a tiny skullcap, this one containing eight electrodes instead of sixteen. After explaining to the mother that we were interested in the changes in the brain associated with different emotions, I asked her to make herself comfortable in front of the TV monitor, holding her baby quietly in her lap. Then I ran the clip.

You might think that inducing a particular emotion in a ten-month-old would be a tricky proposition; all new parents, after all, find themselves dumbstruck as to what makes their babies cry or laugh. But in two important ways babies are actually better test subjects for an experiment like this than my original adults were. First, babies are very expressive emotionally, giggling or crying or recoiling in terror or disgust so strongly that you have no doubt what they're feeling. Also, babies are blissfully ignorant of social constraints. An adult might try to stifle a guffaw if he thinks the humor in a video clip is sophomoric (albeit hilarious) and censor a disgusted grimace if he thinks showing disgust is unmanly. Babies wear their emotions on their sleeves.

The kids didn't let us down. When they saw a video clip of an actress laughing, they smiled—and the left frontal region of their brains crackled with electrical activity. When they watched a clip of an actress sobbing, we immediately had sullen babies on our hands (some even wailed, causing no small amount of consternation in the mothers), and activity in their right prefrontal regions spiked. It really looked as if the left-right pattern of activity underlying positive or negative emotions was present early in life. The study was published in *Science*, and with this, the field of affective neuroscience—the study of the brain basis of emotion—was launched.

Having now seen this left-equals-positive-emotions and right-equals-negative-emotions pattern in ten-month-olds, we wondered if it was there from birth or developed over the first ten months of life. To definitively resolve this question, we had to test newborns. Fortunately, Nathan's lab at Roosevelt Hospital was literally twenty-five steps from the labor and delivery rooms. We therefore stalked the corridors, ambushing new parents (politely—I'd amble up to a father coming for a visit or a mother getting some exercise and ask if they'd be interested in participating in our study). To my surprise, we signed up thirty-three families with no trouble.

We couldn't run videos for newborns; neither their eyesight nor their attention was up to the job of watching. We needed something else that would provoke a clearly positive or negative emotional response. And then I remembered Darwin. In his *Expression of the Emotions in Man and Animals*, he posited that the sense of disgust originates in the rejection of noxious substances from the mouth. I realized we should use tastes. So after a baby had been fed in the nursery (this was back in the day when newborns were kept in a nursery behind those big glass windows you see in old movies) and was quiet but alert, we swooped down and brought him to Nathan's nearby lab. We quickly put on a newborn-size electrode cap and, one by one, dabbed a few drops of distilled water, then sugar water, then lemon juice on his little tongue.

The results were almost comical. The plain water elicited little response, but the sugar water made the babies' faces light up and produced what was very likely their first grin. The lemon juice made them pucker, their eyes squinting and the corners of their mouths drawn back. And to our delight, the

EEGs matched: greater left-side prefrontal activation in response to the sugar water and greater right-side activation in response to the lemon juice. Even though the prefrontal cortex is still very immature at birth, it shows functional differences associated with positive and negative emotions right from the start.

You might be wondering whether these different levels of brain activity—between left and right prefrontal within one person, between one person and another's activity in the left (or right) prefrontal—have anything to do with the real world of how people behave. Good question. Whenever you do a lab experiment in psychology, you worry that the situation is so artificial that it might be irrelevant to how people behave in real life. You also wonder whether your volunteers will figure out what you're attempting to measure and somehow try to manipulate the results. For instance, if they think you're trying to identify what aspects of personality influence whether someone will be a Good Samaritan, volunteers might start acting like Mother Theresa. Or, your volunteers might be lying to you. Maybe they say they're inspired by the clip you just showed them of Martin Luther King Jr.'s "I have a dream" speech, and so you correlate their brain activity with the feeling of being inspired—but in fact the volunteers actually found the clip boring. Unbeknownst to you, you just found the neural correlate of boredom and mislabeled it the neural correlate of inspiration.

Thank God for babies. They can't figure out the actual purpose of your experiment and are far too innocent to lie about what they're experiencing. I mentioned our first babies study, in which Nathan Fox and I found elevated left prefrontal activity when they watched an actress smiling and elevated right prefrontal activity when they watched an actress crying. I assumed that the kids were actually feeling happy or sad. But of course they couldn't tell us. Just to be sure I was right in my inference, I decided to see how babies actually *behaved*.

By this time I was at the University of Wisconsin, Madison, a move I'll recount soon, and my research was entering a new phase. Rather than focusing on general patterns of brain activity accompanying emotions, I began trying to assess the neural basis for individual differences. Up until now I had been looking for patterns that applied to everyone. But as I said in the first chapter, people are very different in how they experience and express emotions. I wanted to see if I could discover a brain basis for those differences, starting with babies.

To recruit ten-month-olds, we used a registry of babies born in the area based upon birth announcements in newspapers. Subjects came to my lab one by one, and after I explained the setup to each mother, I fitted the usual electrode-packed cap over the baby's skull and measured the baseline brain activity. Then I had the mother put her baby in an infant seat and sit beside her child. Once they were settled I told the mother that about ten minutes into the experiment I would give her a sign (a flash of light) that only she would see, which was her cue to get up and leave the room. That's when we started videotaping the abandoned baby. I was interested in seeing whether the baseline measures of brain activity that we had recorded would predict the baby's behavior in response to the separation.

Fortunately for us, the babies were not exactly creative in how they responded to their mothers' departure: They either began wailing almost immediately or appeared very curious and looked around the room with little sign of distress. The measures of baseline brain activity predicted these responses perfectly. The distraught, crying infants had higher baseline levels of right prefrontal activation than did the infants who took their abandonment in stride. This convinced me that baseline measures of brain activity were reflecting something real enough to translate into behavioral differences.

A Depressed Brain

You may recall that Gainotti's patients with damage to their left prefrontal regions experienced pathological crying as well as several classic symptoms of depression. That led to an obvious question: Do patients suffering from depression have diminished activity in their left prefrontal cortex? To find out, I conducted my first study in what would be a long series of experiments on depression and the brain. While still at SUNY Purchase, in the early 1980s, I recruited six people with depression and nine healthy volunteers for a small pilot study. I decided to record baseline brain activity ("baseline" meaning in the absence of any stimulus), during which volunteers were not being instructed to do anything in particular, such as watch a video clip, but to simply "rest" with their eyes open in some periods and closed in others. Presto: Individuals with depressive symptoms had significantly less activation in the left frontal region compared with nondepressed participants.

You would be right in feeling skeptical about a study of only fifteen people, and if the findings came out of the blue and made no physiological sense (for example, a claim that people with depression have very low activity in their visual cortex), your skepticism would be well justified. But despite its limitations, this study was important for several reasons. First, it confirmed in anatomically healthy people (those without brain damage) findings in patients with brain damage (Gainotti's stroke patients): In each case, low levels of activity in the left frontal region of the brain were associated with depression or pathological crying. Second, it suggested that the left prefrontal region contributes something quite specific to our emotional life, namely, positive emotion and the ability to hold in mind a desired goal and form a plan of action to reach it. The lack of these two components is a striking symptom in depression: Many patients report that the absence of joy is even more painful than the presence of sadness, and the inability to engage in goal-directed activity is among the most crippling manifestations of the disease.

Let me recap where things stood. First, when healthy adults experience positive or negative emotion, the left or right side, respectively, of their prefrontal cortex becomes active. Second, the same pattern occurs in babies. Third, depressed patients have a dearth of activity in the left prefrontal cortex or an increase in activity in the right prefrontal, or both.

These results spurred me to wonder if there was a forest around these three trees. In particular, I wondered if what we had identified in the prefrontal cortex might be the neural correlates of approach- and avoidance-related emotion in humans. "Approach" and "avoidance" sound fairly blah, but there is a good case to be made that every emotion we experience falls, at least to some extent, into one or the other of these two categories. (In fact, the great comparative psychologist T. C. Schneirla, whom Jerry Kagan first introduced me to, made exactly this case: Whether to approach or avoid is the fundamental psychological decision an organism makes in relation to its environment.) In this instance, positive emotions with a strong approach component, such as waiting for a loved one to get off a Jetway and then running toward and embracing her, as we used to be able to do before the post-9/11 security precautions, would be associated with activation of the left prefrontal region. Avoidance, such as looking away from a horrific accident scene or cowering in fear at the sound of an intruder in your home, would be associated with activation of the right prefrontal.

Why would evolution have segregated approach and avoidance functions in different hemispheres? It might have something to do with minimizing competition or confusion between them. When we must avoid a harmful or threatening stimulus, it is important that nothing get in the way of our escaping a rock slide or cave bear. Evolution seems to do this by keeping the competing behavior—approach—way over on the other side of the brain, where there is almost no chance it will be activated by mistake.

Individual Differences

You may have noticed that in several of the key studies that launched me on my quest to understand the brain bases of emotion—healthy adults imagining a positive or negative emotional scene, babies watching actresses smile or cry, and newborns tasting sweet and bitter—I compared two or more emotional states and studied the neural differences between them. The first of these experiments was published in 1976. But it was only in 1989, when I was reviewing the raw data from those studies for a book chapter I was writing, that I realized I had missed something profoundly important. There are all sorts of ways one can analyze data, and for the chapter I decided to draw a chart showing the differences in brain activity when my healthy volunteers watched positive- or negative-emotion-inducing video clips. The first time through, I had focused on the fact that when people saw frightening or disgusting clips, activity in the right prefrontal cortex was greater than in the left, and when they watched amusing or uplifting videos, activity was greater in the left than in the right prefrontal. This was the average response for the more than one hundred participants we tested in the different studies.

Now, imagine a bunch of pairs of dots for, say, an amusing clip, one dot way up the graph paper indicating activity in the left prefrontal and one dot way down on the paper showing the very low activity in the right prefrontal. Now imagine a line connecting the two. I drew such lines, in different colors, for each of the participants in our studies. Although what initially caught my eye was the gap between the high dot and the low one, this time I noticed something else. The high dots were not all at the same altitude. The level of activity in one person's left prefrontal cortex when he watched a hilarious clip was immensely higher than that of another person's left prefrontal watching the same clip. Similarly, the level of activity in one person's right prefrontal cortex when she watched a disgusting clip was dramatically lower than in the right prefrontal of another person watching the clip. While activity in the left brain might be 30 percent higher than activity in the right brain (of the same person) when watching a hilarious clip, the difference *between* individuals was as great as 3,000 percent. Some people were off-the-chart happy—if we take "happy" to be quantified by activity in the left prefrontal region.

This was my first glimpse of the dramatic differences between people in terms of how they react to life's experiences (okay, to going into a lab and watching video clips that elicit emotion), with those differences reflected in patterns of brain activity. This is when the idea of Emotional Style was born.

CHAPTER 3

■ ■ ■

Assessing Your Emotional Style

In the introduction, I presented the bare bones of the six elements, or dimensions, that constitute Emotional Style. I imagine that as I asked whether you are the kind of person who can shrug off a minor spat with your spouse, who understands her own emotional state, who can keep his attention focused, and the like, you tried to place yourself along the spectrum of each dimension of Emotional Style. Now I want to be more methodical about it, explaining each dimension in greater depth and offering a way for you to assess your own overall Emotional Style, the product of where you fall on each of the six dimensions. Some of the assessments require nothing more than being insightful and honest about your own behavior and feelings. Others do not lend themselves as readily to self-evaluation, but rather than send you to a psychology lab and a neuroimaging center, I'll offer some next-best ways for you to get a handle on where you fall in these difficult-to-assess dimensions. You can also use the assessments to determine where someone close to you falls on the dimensions; the better you know someone, the more accurate your evaluation is likely to be. Similarly, after you answer each questionnaire about yourself, ask someone close to you to answer them about you. That can serve as a reality check: If someone who knows you very well has very different answers about—to jump ahead here—how long a disagreement leaves you out of sorts, it's a tip-off that you may not be answering correctly or honestly. In each case, I'll start with questions or descriptions about situations that arise in everyday life to get your thoughts going.

The Resilience Dimension

If you have an argument with a friend, does it cast a pall on the remainder of your day? If you arrive at the airport and discover that your flight was canceled, do you sputter profanities at the gate agent, snap at your spouse, feel as if these things always happen to you—and find it impossible to regain your calm and composure for hours? If the vending machine eats your money without giving you the bag of chips, do you pound and yell at the stupid thing, fume for the rest of the day, and give it a surreptitious kick the next time you walk by? If someone close to you dies, do you experience not merely normal sadness but a prolonged and profound despair so debilitating that you are unable to function for months or years? If any or all of these apply to you, then you fall toward the Slow to Recover pole of the Resilience dimension. This part of the continuum is marked by difficulty shaking off anger, sadness, or other negative emotion after a loss, hassle, setback, or other upsetting event.

Alternatively, can you usually brush off setbacks, so when something bad happens you're able to move on? If you argue with your spouse before leaving for work, can you put it behind you with the confidence that it will get resolved? People toward this extreme are Fast to Recover, or resilient.

Either extreme of the dimension can trip you up. An extremely resilient person can lack the motivation to overcome challenges, accepting every setback with a metaphorical shrug and an attitude of "don't worry, be happy." In contrast, being Slow to Recover can prevent you from moving forward after a setback, causing you to continue to fume and obsess over something that is over and done with.

All the examples above—from minor hassles such as the larcenous vending machine to profound losses such as the death of a spouse—have what's called a normative recovery time, the average period it takes to recover. Returning to your baseline emotional state after a death obviously takes longer than regaining your emotional equilibrium after failing to get potato chips from a machine. But no matter how great or small the specific adversity, there are big differences in how quickly people recover. Curiously, perhaps, we are not necessarily conscious of how rapidly we recover, even though the after-shocks of a setback affect our stress levels and mood. You might be irritable for a whole day after a morning argument with a coworker but not realize that your funk is the result of being Slow to Recover. (This ability to introspect and understand our own emotions is an aspect of the Self-Awareness dimension of Emotional Style, described below.)

How quickly or slowly you recover from the setbacks life deals you is in part automatic. When you are flooded with negative emotions, your brain and body immediately activate mechanisms to dampen the emotion and return you to your baseline mood. This happens with positive emotions, too: If that vending machine gives you two bags of chips, the little thrill of pleasure eventually dissipates. In fact, we can measure this recovery time in the laboratory. In a typical experiment, we show volunteers something that makes most people feel sadness, disgust, or another negative emotion, such as pictures of a widow and young children in tears at a funeral or of someone injured in a horrific car accident. Alternatively, we administer a physically painful stimulus, typically via a thermode, a wandlike device filled with very hot water that, when it touches the skin, feels like a hot plate but does not cause any damage.

We then examine what happens in what should be a "recovery period," when the negative feeling or the burning sensation dissipates. For instance, we measure the eyeblink reflex. This is a milder version of the startle reflex, in which suddenly hearing a sharp, loud noise such as a car backfiring or a gunshot can make you jump. With a milder stimulus—we use white noise that sounds like a burst of static on the radio—most people simply blink involuntarily. By measuring (with electrodes) the strength of contraction of the muscle that produces the blink, we can quantify the size of the eyeblink reflex. The blink reflex relates to recovery from an emotional setback: When someone experiences a negative emotion, such as the disgust felt upon seeing a mangled body in a car crash, and then hears the unexpected noise, the eyeblink becomes stronger.

We can use this fact to track what happens in the time after someone has looked at the upsetting photos. By presenting the startling noise in the first few seconds after the person sees the photos, then again thirty seconds after, and finally one minute after, measuring the blink reflex each time, we can track how rapidly someone recovers from the negative emotion by determining when the strength of the person's eyeblink reflex returns to what it was before exposure to the disturbing photos. The faster the recovery, the more resilient the person is in the face of adversity. It turns out that the very short time scale in the laboratory experiment is related to the much longer time scale for real-life events, so although we are measuring recovery periods in seconds, they predict the much longer recovery periods of real life, which take minutes or hours or more.

I don't recommend trying this at home; for one thing, the equipment to measure the strength of the eye-contracting muscles isn't something you can buy at the local hardware store. But to get a sense of your Resilience, the next best thing is to ask yourself the following questions. Answer each one True or False. If you are tempted to think long and hard about a question, or if you feel that there are too many nuances and exceptions, resist. The most accurate results come from making a snap judgment about whether a question is True or False about you. If you do not want to write in the book (or if you are reading this as an e-book or listening to the audio version), just grab some scrap paper, scribble "Resilience" across the top, and write the numbers 1 through 10 down the side. Write True or False for each question. I'll tell you how to score your answers at the end of the questionnaire. You can do basically the same thing for each of the other five questionnaires.

1. If I have a minor disagreement with a close friend or spouse—
   closer to "No, it's *your* turn to do the dishes" than *"You cheated
   on me?!"*—it typically leaves me out of sorts for hours or longer.

2. If another driver uses the shoulder to zoom up to the front of a
   long line of traffic waiting to merge, I am likely to shake it off
   easily rather than fume about it for a long time.

3. When I have experienced profound grief, such as the death of
   someone close to me, it has interfered with my ability to function for many months.

4. If I make a mistake at work and get reprimanded for it, I can
   shrug it off and take it as a learning experience.

5. If I try a new restaurant and find that the food is awful and the service snooty, it ruins my whole evening.

6. If I'm stuck in traffic because of an accident up ahead, when I pass the bottleneck I typically floor it to vent my frustration but still seethe inside.

7. If my home's water heater breaks, it does not affect my mood very much, since I know I can just call a plumber and get it fixed.

8. If I meet a wonderful man/woman and ask if he/she would like to get together again, being told no typically puts me in a bad mood for hours or even days.

9. If I am being considered for an important professional award or promotion and it goes to someone I consider less qualified, I can usually move on quickly.

10. At a party, if I'm having a conversation with an interesting stranger and get completely tongue-tied when he/she asks me about myself, I tend to replay the conversation—this time including what I *should* have said—for hours or even days afterward.

You may have noticed that the questions cover a broad range of setbacks, from the trivial (question 5, for instance) to the profound (question 3). That's intentional. My research has consistently demonstrated that recovery from the minor challenges we administer in an experiment, such as being burned by the thermode or seeing an upsetting picture, is strongly correlated with and predictive of how someone copes with real-life adversity, particularly how quickly they recover. Resilience on the little things is therefore a good indicator of Resilience on bigger ones. While it is true that some people actually enjoy obsessing over small setbacks but can step up to the plate in a real emergency, their Resilience in each situation is likely to be the same: If they recover quickly from the little setbacks, they tend to be resilient in the face of big ones, and if they become paralyzed by or obsess over the little things, they tend to be laid low for a long time by the big things, too.

Give yourself one point for each True answer to questions 1, 3, 5, 6, 8, and 10; give yourself zero points for each False answer. Give yourself one point for each False answer to questions 2, 4, 7, and 9; score zero points for each True answer. Anything above seven suggests you are Slow to Recover. If you scored below three, you are Fast to Recover and thus quite resilient.

To better understand people close to you, you might also ask yourself the above questions about them. Similarly, you can have someone who knows you well answer these questions about you. Sometimes, other people see us more clearly than we see ourselves. You may answer with an emphatic *no* the questions about whether a minor setback leaves you fuming for the rest of the day, but your significant other might disagree.

The Outlook Dimension

We all know the type: She charges into gatherings where she doesn't know a soul and manages to connect with perfect strangers. He has never let an emotional cloud darken his sunny outlook on life. She maintains a high level of energy and engagement even in the most trying circumstances. He delights in every social encounter, rather than viewing it as a trial. She feels a sense of interconnectedness with her surroundings, both social and natural. He derives unvarnished pleasure from a life that, objectively, could easily be a source of unhappiness or anxiety. These kinds of people seem to see a silver lining in every cloud. They're the ones we sometimes want to shake, screaming, "Don't you see the world is going to hell?" Of course they don't; the way their brains work, they see the positive in everything—which can blind them to warning signs in both their personal and their professional lives. These are the people who inhabit the optimistic, Positive extreme of the Outlook dimension. They have an uncanny ability to *maintain* positive emotions. The "maintain" aspect is the key characteristic of this dimension: It measures not whether you can feel joy but how well you can keep that feeling alive.

At the other end of the spectrum are people in whom joy tends to melt away as quickly as a snowflake in the sun. These are the cynics and pessimists who, if they feel an initial jolt of happiness or pride over some encounter or accomplishment, cannot sustain it. Sometimes the inability to sustain a positive emotion is so extreme that they hardly feel it in the first place— "blink and you'll miss it." As a result, people at the extreme Negative pole of this dimension have difficulty experiencing pleasure for any length of time and can be at risk for clinical depression or addiction. They can be described as gloomy, Negative types.

The capacity to remain upbeat and to sustain positive emotion over time is the key measure of the Outlook dimension of your Emotional Style. It can be thought of as the complement to Resilience, which reflects how quickly you recover from adversity. Outlook reflects how long and how well you can sustain positive emotions, either after something good happens to you or as a result of deliberately engaging in emotionally positive thoughts, such as thinking about someone you love. The durability of positive feelings has a strong carryover effect on your overall outlook (hence the name of this dimension): Someone whose positive mood hangs around tends to be optimistic, while someone whose moments of joy can be measured in microseconds feels chronically down and pessimistic.

In the lab, we measure Outlook by observing how long brain circuitry underlying positive emotion remains active when people are shown pictures that activate that circuitry, such as a glowing mother embracing her baby or a Good Samaritan going to the aid of someone in distress. We also measure Outlook by measuring how long facial muscles associated with smiling are activated in response to a stimulus like these. In people who fall at the Positive extreme, brain circuits associated with positive emotion stay active for much longer than they do in people who fall at the Negative end; their smile muscles also remain activated for longer. Again, this isn't something you can try at home. But you can get a sense of whether you tend toward the Positive or Negative end of the Outlook dimension by answering these questions True or False. Again, don't ponder them too long and think of all sorts of exceptions and mitigating circumstances; go with your initial impression.

1. When I am invited to meet new people, I look forward to it, thinking they might become my friends, rather than seeing it as a chore, figuring these people will never be worth knowing.

2. When evaluating a coworker, I focus on details about which areas he needs to improve rather than on his positive overall performance.

3. I believe the next ten years will be better for me than the last ten.

4. Faced with the possibility of moving to a new city, I regard it as a frightening step into the unknown.

5. When something small but unexpected and positive happens to me in the morning—for example, having a great conversation with a stranger—the positive mood fades within minutes.

6. When I go to a party and I'm having a good time at the outset, the positive feeling tends to last for the entire evening.

7. I find that beautiful scenes such as a gorgeous sunset quickly wear off and I get bored easily.

8. When I wake up in the morning I can think of a pleasant activity that I've planned, and the thought puts me in a good mood that lasts the entire day.

9. When I go to a museum or attend a concert, the first few minutes are really enjoyable, but it doesn't last.

10. I often feel that on busy days I can keep going from one event to the next without getting tired.

If the questions seem to cover your disposition about the future as well as your ability to maintain a positive feeling about an event in the past, that's intentional: The Outlook dimension of Emotional Style captures both. And as was the case with Resilience, your Outlook about trivial events is correlated with and predictive of your Outlook about momentous ones. Although individual circumstances will affect the answers—it is easier for a twentysomething single to move to a new city than it is for a fortysomething with a spouse and children who would need to adapt to new schools—the questions nevertheless capture the core of the Outlook dimension.

Give yourself one point for each True answer to questions 1, 3, 6, 8, and 10; score zero for each False answer. Give yourself one point for each False answer to 2, 4, 5, 7, and 9; score zero for each True answer. The higher your score, the closer you are to the Positive end of the Outlook style. Anything above seven is a Positive type, while a score below three is a Negative type.

The Social Intuition Dimension

You've probably seen it: A man and a woman are talking, and he looks away, leans back, takes half a step away from her... and still she has no idea that he has absolutely no interest in her. Or maybe you have had a friend grab you as you're dashing out the door in a rush, and he begins jabbering away about a long and complicated experience he wants your advice on—while the whole time you're inching toward your car and checking your watch. And still he won't let you go. People at this extreme on the Social Intuition spectrum are Puzzled.

At the other extreme are Socially Intuitive types. They have an uncanny ability to pick up on subtle nonverbal cues, to read other people's body language, vocal intonation, and facial expressions. They can tell when someone who is grieving wants to talk about her loss and when she wants to be distracted by gossip and chitchat. They can tell when a colleague who has been reprimanded by a supervisor wants advice and consolation and when he wants to be left alone. They can tell when a child who has suffered his first romantic rejection wants advice about relationships and when he wants them to pretend they have no idea what's going on.

People differ dramatically in how attuned they are to nonverbal social cues. Extreme insensitivity to these signals is characteristic of people on the autism spectrum, who struggle to read facial expressions and other social cues, but people who fall well short of a clinical diagnosis can also be socially deaf and blind, with devastating consequences for personal and professional relationships. Conversely, acute sensitivity to the emotional state of others is central to both empathy and compassion, since being able to decode and understand social signals means we can respond to them.

Indeed, Social Intuition is the hallmark of some of our greatest teachers, therapists, and others in the caring professions. The Dalai Lama has it in abundance. A few years ago he was visiting a meditation center in western Massachusetts. Everyone there was abuzz with excitement, especially the cofounder—who, a week before, had broken her leg and had to get around on crutches. While more than a hundred people stood outside the main building waiting to greet the Dalai Lama as he arrived, she stood all the way at the back of the crowd. She had never met him and was feeling very disappointed, thinking her leg would keep her from doing so. When the Dalai Lama emerged from the car, he looked at the crowd and somehow noticed the woman way in back. Deploying his social antennae, he politely weaved his way through the clusters of people directly to her and asked, "What happened? Are you okay?" And with that, he made her feel that she was, at least at that moment, the center of his universe.

I have often been the fortunate beneficiary of the Dalai Lama's Social Intuition. In 2010, at the end of a meeting he had held for scientists and Buddhist scholars, he turned to me to say good-bye and suddenly grabbed me in a bear hug. "I know that we were together in a former life," he said—the highest praise one could imagine from the spiritual head of Tibetan Buddhism. A few months before, when the Dalai Lama attended the inauguration of the University of Wisconsin's Center for Investigating Healthy Minds, which I direct, a number of dignitaries had been invited to attend a lunch hosted by the university chancellor. We thought the Dalai Lama would be more comfortable having a lunch of Tibetan food with Buddhist monks he was traveling with, but when he saw the small group he asked, "Where is everyone else?" Learning that the chancellor's bash was a few buildings away, he told Tenzin Takla, his chief of staff, "I'd like to go there." Now, for the Dalai Lama to go anywhere in the United States is no simple thing, especially when it deviates from an agreed-upon plan. As he strode toward the exit, intent on going to the chancellor's, all of the intimidating-looking guys with earpieces—that would be the Secret Service protection that the U.S. government always provides—looked like they were going to have heart attacks. They barked orders into their headsets, repositioned the FBI snipers on surrounding rooftops, and off we went. When the Dalai Lama got to the chancellor's, where I tried to usher him to a quiet table and get waiters to bring him lunch, he would have none of it. Maroon robe swirling, he walked up to the buffet table, took a plate, and waited in line to serve himself like everyone else—attracting no small number of stares but even more smiles of appreciation that this Nobel laureate, head of the Tibetan government in exile, best-selling author, and spiritual leader was waiting his turn for poached salmon, rice pilaf, and a Weight Watchers nightmare of desserts like everyone else. Social Intuition, indeed.

In the lab, we assess Social Intuition through measurements of both brain function and behavior. When we show someone a picture of a face, for instance, we use special laser eye-tracking devices to measure where his eyes are actually looking. Someone who looks at the eye region of the face tends to have stronger Social Intuition than someone who looks at the mouth, and someone who looks away tends to have poor Social Intuition. If we use the laser device when someone is having her brain scanned by fMRI, we can measure brain activity simultaneously. We look for activation in the fusiform gyrus, which is part of the visual cortex, and the amygdalae, key structures in a circuit known to be important for social cognition. (The brain has two amygdalae, little almond-shaped bodies buried within the temporal lobes on each side of the brain. From now on, I will use the singular, amygdala, to refer to the pair.) These regions are typically activated when you process another person's face and especially when you look at the person's eyes, which convey a significant amount of emotional information.

To gauge where you fall on the spectrum of Social Intuition, answer these questions True or False.

1. When I'm talking with people, I often notice subtle social cues about their emotions—discomfort, say, or anger—before they acknowledge those feelings in themselves.
2. I often find myself noting facial expressions and body language.
3. I find it does not really matter if I talk with people on the phone or in person, since I rarely get any additional information from seeing whom I'm speaking with.
4. I often feel as though I know more about people's true feelings than they do themselves.
5. I am often taken by surprise when someone I'm talking with gets angry or upset at something I said, for no apparent reason.
6. At a restaurant, I prefer to sit next to someone I'm speaking with so I don't have to see his or her full face.
7. I often find myself responding to another person's discomfort or distress on the basis of an intuitive feel rather than an explicit discussion.
8. When I am in public places with time to kill, I like to observe people around me.

9.   I find it uncomfortable when someone I barely know looks directly into my eyes during a conversation.

10. I can often tell when something is bothering another person just by looking at him or her.

Give yourself one point for each True answer for questions 1, 2, 4, 7, 8, and 10; score one point for each False answer for questions 3, 5, 6, and 9. Score zero for each False answer to 1, 2, 4, 7, 8, and 10, and for each True answer to 3, 5, 6, and 9. The higher your score (eight or above), the more Socially Intuitive you are; a lower score (three or below) means you are closer to Puzzled.

The Self-Awareness Dimension

Do you have friends for whom introspection seems as foreign as Urdu? Do you yourself act and react without knowing why, as if your inner self is opaque to your consciousness, an utter mystery? Do those closest to you ask why you seem anxious, jealous, angry, or impatient—and now that it's been called to your attention, are you surprised that you do feel that way? We have all known people who are completely blind and deaf to their own emotions. They're not in denial; they are honestly unaware of emotional cues that arise within their own bodies. In part, that reflects differences in the strength of such signals. But it also reflects differences in the ability to recognize and interpret those signals, as well as sensitivity to them (that is, how strong the signals must be in order for you to perceive them). Some people have a very hard time "feeling" their feelings: It may take them days to recognize that they're angry, sad, jealous, or afraid. At this extreme of the Self-Awareness dimension are people who are Self-Opaque.

At the other end are Self-Aware people, who are acutely conscious of their thoughts and feelings and attuned to the messages their body sends them. They know that the real reason they're yelling at the kids is not that refusing to eat kale is so heinous, but that a monster traffic jam on the way home put them an hour behind schedule for the evening, ratcheting up their stress level to TILT. They can be supersensitive to the messages their body transmits, experiencing the physical aspects of their emotional states with heightened, sometimes crippling intensity. This heightened sensitivity can be beneficial in several ways. It appears to play a crucial role in empathy, the ability to feel what others are feeling, and by allowing you to understand your own emotional state it can help you avoid misunderstandings during arguments with a significant other: If you grasp that you are upset about something that happened before you got home, then you are more likely to understand that the explosive anger you are suddenly feeling is not really because dinner isn't on the table yet.

High Self-Awareness can also exact a cost, however. Someone with very sensitive emotional antennae for his own feelings who observes the pain of another will feel that person's anxiety or sadness in both mind and body—experiencing a surge of the stress hormone cortisol, for instance, as well as elevated heart rate and blood pressure. Such extreme sensitivity is likely a factor in the burnout that nurses, counselors, therapists, and social workers suffer.

In the lab, one way we measure people's sensitivity to their internal physiological signals is by how well they can detect their own heartbeat. First, we measure a person's heart rate while she is resting comfortably. Then we use a computer to construct a series of ten tones perfectly in sync with her heartbeat; each tone occurs precisely when the heart beats. We then construct a second sequence, shifted a bit, so that the tones sound a little before or after each heartbeat. To assess how sensitive the person is to her internal signals, we play (through headphones) two sequences of ten tones; her task is to choose which one is in sync with her heartbeat. We run the in-sync and out-of-sync sequences a hundred or so times each, alternating them randomly. Self-Aware people score in the top 25 percent of performance on this test.

Assessing your sensitivity to your body's signals doesn't lend itself to the kind of questionnaire we've developed for the other five dimensions of Emotional Style, so I've included both questions and a simple exercise you can try. The latter should be done with a partner.

1. Often, when someone asks me why I am so angry or sad, I respond (or think to myself), "But I'm not!"
2. When those closest to me ask why I treated someone brusquely or meanly, I often disagree that I did any such thing.

3. I frequently—more than a couple of times a month—find that my heart is racing or my pulse is pounding, and I have no idea why.

4. When I observe someone in pain, I feel the pain myself both emotionally and physically.

5. I am usually sure enough about how I am feeling that I can put my emotions into words.

6. I sometimes notice aches and pains and have no idea where they came from.

7. I like to spend time being quiet and relaxed, just feeling what is going on inside me.

8. I believe I very much inhabit my body and feel at home and comfortable with my body.

9. I am strongly oriented to the external world and rarely take note of what's happening in my body.

10. When I exercise, I am very sensitive to the changes it produces in my body.

Give yourself one point for each True response to questions 4, 5, 7, 8, and 10; score one point for each False response to questions 1, 2, 3, 6, and 9. Score zero for each False response to 4, 5, 7, 8, and 10, and for each True response to 1, 2, 3, 6, and 9. A score of eight or higher means you are Self-Aware; a score below three means you are Self-Opaque.

For the exercise, have a partner take your pulse for thirty seconds while you direct your attention internally and try to detect your own heartbeat. Focus your awareness on your internal bodily sensations, and do your best (without touching your wrist or anyplace else to feel a pulse) to sense your heartbeat and count the number of beats. Do this three more times—that is, four thirty-second trials. Compare your counts to those of your partner. The closer the match, the greater your Self-Awareness.

The Sensitivity to Context Dimension

Have you ever told your boss the same dirty joke you told your friends at the sports bar the night before? Have you ever been at a funeral and been appalled to see someone playing Angry Birds on his iPhone? How about being at a wedding where another guest regales the table with an account of her long-ago affair with the groom? Are you baffled when people tell you that your behavior is inappropriate?

Most of us know when conversations with a particular emotional tinge have no place in a given circumstance. People who are especially aware of the social surround are at the Tuned In pole of the Sensitivity to Context spectrum. People who are oblivious to the social surround fall at the Tuned Out extreme: They're oblivious to the implicit rules that govern social interactions and that make a behavior that would be perfectly acceptable in one context offensive in another. Because sensitivity to context is largely intuitive rather than something we consciously regulate, and because both social context and our own behavior frequently have emotional subtexts (wedding: happy, decorous; affair with groom: tawdry), I consider it an important component of Emotional Style.

Depending on whom we are interacting with and in what circumstances, there are different rules and expectations—for interactions with close friends, people you know only slightly, family members, coworkers, or superiors. Nothing good can come of treating your boss like a child, or of treating the cop who just pulled you over like a drinking buddy, let alone treating a coworker like a lover. Sensitivity to the rules of social engagement and the capacity to regulate our emotions and behavior accordingly varies enormously among people. You can think of the Sensitivity to Context dimension of Emotional Style as the outer-directed version of the Self-Awareness style: Just as the latter reflects how attuned you are to your own physiological and emotional cues, so Sensitivity to Context reflects how attuned you are to the social environment.

In the lab, we measure this dimension by determining how emotional behavior varies with social context. For example, toddlers tend to be wary in unfamiliar circumstances such as a lab but not in a familiar environment. A toddler who seems perpetually wary at home is therefore probably insensitive to context. For adults, we test Sensitivity to Context by conducting the first round of tests in one room and then a second round in a different room. By determining to what extent emotional responses vary by the environment in which testing occurs, we can infer how keenly someone perceives and feels the effects of context. We also make brain measurements: The hippocampus appears to play an especially important role in apprehending context, so we measure hippocampal function and structure with MRI.

To get a sense of where you fall on the Sensitivity to Context spectrum, answer True or False to these questions:

1. I have been told by someone close to me that I am unusually sensitive to other people's feelings.
2. I have occasionally been told that I behaved in a socially inappropriate way, which surprised me.
3. I have sometimes suffered a setback at work or had a falling-out with a friend because I was too chummy with a superior or too jovial when a good friend was distraught.
4. When I speak with people, they sometimes move back to increase the distance between us.
5. I often find myself censoring what I was about to say because I've sensed something in the situation that would make it inappropriate (e.g., before I respond to, "Honey, do these jeans make me look fat?").
6. When I am in a public setting like a restaurant, I am especially aware of modulating how loudly I speak.
7. I have frequently been reminded when in public to avoid mentioning the names of people who might be around.
8. I am almost always aware of whether I have been someplace before, even if it is a highway that I last drove many years ago.
9. I notice when someone is acting in a way that seems out of place, such as behaving too casually at work.
10. I've been told by those close to me that I show good manners with strangers and in new situations.

Give yourself one point for each True answer to questions 1, 5, 6, 8, 9, and 10; score one point for each False answer to questions 2, 3, 4, and 7. Score zero for each False answer to 1, 5, 6, 8, 9, and 10, and for each True answer to 2, 3, 4, and 7. If you scored below three, you fall at the Tuned Out end of the spectrum, while a score of eight or above indicates you are very Tuned In to context.

The Attention Dimension

Can you screen out emotional distractions and stay focused? Or do your thoughts flit from the task at hand to the fight you had with your spouse that morning, the anxiety you feel about an upcoming presentation for work, or the follow-up medical appointment you have tomorrow? If you're rushing to meet a deadline and your boss appears at your elbow every half hour to see how you're doing, does it take you several minutes after she leaves to regain your train of thought? How about after your teenager calls about his latest college-application crisis? (A school that won't accept the common-application essay?!)

It may seem odd to include attention as a dimension of Emotional Style, since the ability to focus attention is usually thought of as a component of cognitive ability. The reason I include it is that while plain old sights and sounds are distracting enough, when they come with an emotional overlay they can be even more so. In a noisy restaurant, for instance, if we hear shouting a few tables away, or perhaps a loud and agitated voice followed by the sound of glass shattering, it is more difficult to remain focused on our conversation than when the surrounding voices are less emotionally laden.

Emotional cues are not only ubiquitous in our lives and environment, they are also strong distractions, often interfering with our ability to both accomplish tasks and maintain equanimity. It turns out that the ability to screen out emotional distractions is correlated with the ability to screen out sensory distractions. A Focused person can zoom in on a single conversation at a noisy party, while an Unfocused one is constantly shifting her attention and her eyes to the most attention-grabbing stimulus. Some people can plug away despite being in the throes of emotional turmoil; they fall at the Focused extreme of the Attention spectrum. Others are constantly distracted by emotional impulses that have nothing to do with the task at hand; they fall at the Unfocused extreme. Focused people can concentrate despite emotion-laden intrusions, filtering out the anxiety supercharging the air around them, while the Unfocused cannot. In short, attention and emotion are intimate partners. Since emotional stimuli command an untoward share of our attention, maintaining a stable internal compass that allows us to calmly focus and resist distractions is an aspect of Emotional Style.

In many ways, being able to screen out emotional distractions provides the building blocks for other aspects of our emotional life, in that focused attention plays a role in other dimensions of Emotional Style: Self-Awareness, for instance, requires paying attention to signals from your body, and Social Intuition requires focusing on social cues.

In the lab, we measure Attention in several ways—because, it turns out, there are several distinct forms of attention. One is selective attention. This is the ability to be immersed in the constant sea of stimuli that surrounds us and yet, miraculously, pay attention to only one thing. I say "miraculously" because the amount of information we're exposed to at any moment is staggering. Even as you read these words, your peripheral vision is taking in your hands as they hold the book. Your ears are taking in sounds; if you think you're in a silent room, stop reading and focus on what you can hear. Your feet are pushing against the floor, and your bottom is pushing against a seat; again, stop reading and focus on what your body feels—see what I mean? If you weren't paying attention to any of these things until now, congratulations on a commendable feat of focus. Yet despite all these stimuli competing for our attention, we (often) manage to focus on only one and ignore the others. If we couldn't, we would be hopelessly tossed about in the vast ocean of our sensory world. We manage this focus in two ways: by enhancing the input in the "channel" we want to pay attention to (the words of this sentence) and by inhibiting the input in the ignored channels (what your bottom is feeling, etc.).

Another form of attention is open, nonjudgmental awareness. This is the capacity to remain receptive to whatever might pass into your thoughts, view, hearing, or feeling and to do so in a noncritical way. For instance, if you are aware of a mild pain in your lower back but are able to simply notice it without your thoughts getting hijacked by it, then you are practicing open, nonjudgmental awareness. If you feel a pang of worry about being late for a meeting because the elevator is broken, and you simply tell yourself, "Hmm, I feel myself getting stressed out," but do not panic as you look around for the stairs, then you are practicing open, nonjudgmental awareness. Someone who is skilled at this often seems to have a kind of inner magnet that keeps his focus where he intends and does not let it get pulled hither and yon by events.

This is the kind of awareness that many forms of meditation cultivate, as I'll explain in chapter 9. It generates a sense of contentment and emotional balance (another reason attention is part of Emotional Style); people who fall at the Focused end of the Attention spectrum tend to be unflappable, not pushed and pulled by constant emotional ups and downs. Open, nonjudgmental awareness is also critical for being tuned in to our surroundings as well as our own thoughts and emotions, and as such plays an important role in Self-Awareness and Social Intuition. Without a capacity for open, nonjudgmental awareness, we can miss both subtle cues arising from within our own body and mind and the nuanced cues in our social environment.

To measure open, nonjudgmental awareness in the lab, we start with the fact that if one stimulus hijacks our attention, we won't notice other stimuli that occur just a fraction of a second later. This blindness (or deafness) to subsequent stimuli is called the attentional blink, and there is a simple test that measures it. In one version, you watch as a barrage of letters flashes onto a screen, one after another, ten per second: C, P, Q, D, K, L, T, B, X, V, etc. But every now and then a number appears, as in C, P, Q, D, 3, K, L, 7, T, B, X, V. The task is to indicate when a number interrupts the stream of letters. If the second number follows the first within about half a second or less, most people notice the first number (the 3) but literally do not see the second (the 7). Their attention has blinked. The reason seems to be that, because the numbers appear rarely and because they're your quarry, when one does show up you feel a frisson of excitement; it takes time for the brain to return to a state in which it can perceive its quarry. The longer your attentional blink—that is, the more time you need before you can perceive the next number amid the barrage of letters—the longer it takes your brain to be able to attend to the next stimulus, and the more information you miss in the world around you.

Attentional blinks last even longer when there is an emotional component to what you are supposed to be noticing. In this version of the experiment, instead of watching a series of letters interrupted by an occasional number, volunteers watch for, say, a picture of a crying child amid a stream of outdoor scenes. In this case, the time needed before we are able to perceive another image of a crying child is greater than with letters and numbers, a hint that attention has an emotional component or, more precisely, that emotions affect attention.

Some people, however, have almost no attentional blink. They have a kind of nonreactive awareness that can perceive stimuli with such equanimity that the little thrill the rest of us feel when we perceive a number among the letters is either absent entirely or, if present, doesn't cause their attention to blink. As a result, they tend to miss fewer of the stimuli than the rest of us. The extent to which people blink, particularly with emotional stimuli, reflects a quality of emotional balance and equanimity.

In the lab, we assess open, nonjudgmental awareness through the attentional blink test, using either the letters-and-numbers version or the variation with emotionally laden or nature scenes. We measure focused attention by presenting simple tones of different pitch, typically one high and one low, through earphones. A participant is first asked to pay attention to only the high-pitched tone and to press a button each time she hears it, but not to press when she hears the low-pitched tone. To make the task more difficult, we pipe in the tones separately to either the right or left ear, about once a second, alternating between ears. The participant's score—how many tones she correctly pressed the button for, minus incorrect presses—is a measure of her capacity for focused attention. To ratchet up the difficulty further, we sometimes tell participants to press the button only if they hear the high tone in the left ear, or the low tone in the right ear, or any such combination. Often what happens is that when the high-pitched tone sounds in the unattended ear (the one the person is supposed to ignore), the participant will press the button in error, an indication that his attention is too broad and insufficiently focused. And sometimes he simply misses the presentation of the high-pitched tone. In all these cases, we simultaneously take brain readings with either fMRI or EEG, depending on whether we want to focus on the timing of brain activity (in which case EEG is better) or the location (in which case we use fMRI).

Absent all this equipment, you can assess your Attention style by answering True or False to these statements:

1.   I can concentrate in a noisy environment.
2.   When I am in a situation in which a lot is going on and there is a great deal of sensory stimulation, such as at a party or in a crowd at an airport, I can keep myself from getting lost in a train of thought about any particular thing I see.
3.   If I decide to focus my attention on a particular task, I find that I am mostly able to keep it there.

4. If I am at home and trying to work, the noises of a television or other people make me very distracted.
5. I find that if I sit quietly for even a few moments, a flood of thoughts rush into my mind and I find myself following multiple strands of thought, often without knowing how each one began.
6. If I am distracted by some unexpected event, I can refocus my attention on what I had been doing.
7. During periods of relative quiet, such as when I'm sitting on a train or a bus or waiting in line at a store, I notice a lot of the things around me.
8. When an important solo project requires my full and focused attention, I try to work in the quietest place I can find.
9. My attention tends to get captured by stimuli and events in the environment, and it is difficult for me to disengage once this happens.
10. It is easy for me to talk with another person in a crowded situation like a cocktail party or a cubicle in an office; I can tune out others in such an environment even when, with concentration, I can make out what they are saying.

Give yourself one point for each True answer to questions 1, 2, 3, 6, 7, and 10; score one point for each False answer to questions 4, 5, 8, and 9. Score zero for each False answer to 1, 2, 3, 6, 7, and 10, and for each True answer to 4, 5, 8, and 9. A score of eight or above means you fall at the Focused end of the Attention dimension, while a score of three or below means you tend to be Unfocused.

Now that you have assessed where you fall on each of the six dimensions of Emotional Style, get a piece of paper and draw six horizontal lines, evenly spaced from top to bottom:

- Label the first line Resilience, and continue through Outlook, Social Intuition, Self-Awareness, Sensitivity to Context, and Attention.
- Label each extreme of each dimension, from left to right. For Resilience, the ends are Fast to Recover and Slow to Recover. For

Outlook, Negative and Positive. For Social Intuition, Puzzled and Socially Intuitive. For Self-Awareness, Self-Opaque and Self-Aware. For Sensitivity to Context, Tuned Out and Tuned In. For Attention, Unfocused and Focused.

- Now, depending on what you scored on each of the six questionnaires, make a mark on each line.

You can see at a glance your overall Emotional Style. Maybe you are a sort of Positive person who is Fast to Recover, Socially Intuitive, Self-Opaque, Tuned In, and Focused. Maybe you are Negative but Fast to Recover, Puzzled about the social surround, Self-Opaque, and Unfocused. Whatever your Emotional Style, knowing it is the first step toward understanding how it affects your health and your relationships, and the first step toward deciding if you would like to move it toward the right or the left on any of the six dimensions.

Here is my own Emotional Style diagram:

Resilience
1   2   10
FAST TO RECOVER   SLOW TO RECOVER

Outlook
1   7   10
NEGATIVE   POSITIVE

Social Intuition
1   7   10
PUZZLED   SOCIALLY INTUITIVE

Self-Awareness
1   8   10
SELF-OPAQUE   SELF-AWARE

Sensitivity to Context
1   8   10
TUNED-OUT   TUNED-IN

Attention
1   9   10
UNFOCUSED   FOCUSED

Davidson's scores on the questionnaires assessing Emotional Style.

I explained in the introduction that my focus on the six dimensions of Emotional Style rather than on the better-known types of personality reflects the fact that these six have a solid foundation in patterns of brain activity. In the next chapter, I will explain how we discovered that, what the patterns are, and why they are crucial both to understanding Emotional Style and to contemplating ways to shift it along one or more of the six dimensions.

CHAPTER 4

■ ■ ■

The Brain Basis of Emotional Style

In this era of the brain, when even advertising agencies want to know how consumers' amygdalae react to a commercial, it seems patently obvious that the thoughts we think and the emotions we feel reflect patterns of brain activity. When we conjure up a mental image of our home, we can thank activity in the visual cortex for our ability to see, in our mind's eye, exactly where the mailbox is relative to the front door. When we hear and understand a complex sentence, it's because circuits in our temporal lobe interact with those in the prefrontal cortex to pull meaning from the auditory signals. When we plan a vacation and mentally rehearse getting everyone to the airport, we draw upon the huge expanse of the prefrontal cortex, a time machine that has the power to transport our thoughts into the future.

So, too, with the six dimensions of Emotional Style: They reflect activity in specific, identifiable brain circuits. Each dimension has two extremes, such as Positive and Negative in the case of Outlook, which are usually the result of heightened or reduced activity in those circuits. The first step to understanding why you are the way you are, as indicated in the drawing you made of your results on the questionnaires in the previous chapter, is therefore understanding the brain basis for each dimension and for the extremes of each. This is also the first step toward nudging yourself in either direction along any of the dimensions. I am, admittedly, biased, but I believe that any program that purports to alter something as fundamental as Emotional Style simply has greater credibility if it is grounded in neuroscience.

It's hardly surprising that where you fall on each dimension of Emotional Style is the result of specific patterns of brain activity, since everything in our mental life is. What is surprising, however, is that much of the circuitry underlying the six dimensions lies far from the brain's supposed emotion regions—the limbic system and the hypothalamus. This emerged from the discovery that started it all: that the prefrontal cortex, site of such executive functions as planning and judgment, controls how emotionally resilient people are.

The study that showed this, which I described in chapter 2, was done when I was at SUNY Purchase, but I soon realized that Purchase was too small and lacked the necessary infrastructure for the research I wanted to do. Soon after I began to put out feelers for positions at larger, more research-oriented universities, I heard that Peter Lang, a well-known psychophysiologist, was leaving the University of Wisconsin, Madison, to be with his significant other. Wisconsin decided to replace him with someone who did vaguely similar research, and they approached me. (Wisconsin has a winning strategy for recruiting faculty, recruiting those whose star is still rising rather than going after full-blown supernovas, as a place like Harvard typically does.) They made me an offer and I accepted, in large part because of the stellar reputation of the school's psychology department.

I moved to Madison in September 1985, starting a new job in a new state under less than ideal personal circumstances: My wife, Susan, and three-year-old daughter stayed behind in New York so Susan could complete her residency in obstetrics and gynecology at the Albert Einstein College of Medicine. I found a tiny apartment with a beat-up sofa bed, and for the first year I commuted between time zones, spending Thursday through Sunday nights in New York and flying to Madison very early each Monday morning. My resilient, positive-outlook Emotional Style definitely helped keep the stress from overwhelming me.

The Resilient Brain

At one end of the Resilience dimension are people who get so beaten down by adversity that they recover very, very slowly or not at all, while at the other extreme are people who either shrug off setbacks and continue on their life's course or actively fight back, thus recovering quickly from adversity. As I described in chapter 2, Resilience is marked by greater left versus right activation in the prefrontal cortex, while a lack of Resilience comes from higher right prefrontal activation. The amount of activation in the left prefrontal region of a Resilient person can be thirty times that in someone who is not Resilient.

This was the first hint that different levels of activity in a specific brain region determine where someone falls on one dimension of Emotional Style. Intriguing as this was, I didn't want to go out on a limb with a claim about the brain basis for individual differences unless I knew it wasn't going to crack beneath me and send my nascent career plunging into early ignominy. The study that revealed the left-right prefrontal difference was pretty small (only a few dozen subjects), and the difference emerged in only the one protocol that we used—showing people emotional video clips. Obviously, I needed more solid evidence. Once I was at Madison, I therefore began to reflect more deeply on what the variations in patterns of prefrontal function might mean and, in particular, to ask what the prefrontal cortex does in emotion. After all, the prefrontal cortex was, and is, known to be the site of the highest of higher-order cognitive activity, the seat of judgment and planning and other executive functions. How could it possibly play a role in a key element of *Emotional Style?*

One clue came from the large bundles of neurons running between certain regions of the prefrontal cortex and the amygdala. The amygdala is involved in negative emotion and distress, snapping to attention and activity when we feel anxious, afraid, or threatened. Perhaps, I thought, the left prefrontal cortex might inhibit the amygdala and, through this mechanism, help to facilitate rapid recovery from adversity.

To test this idea, graduate student Daren Jackson and I recruited forty-seven adults with an average age of fifty-eight. They were all part of the Wisconsin Longitudinal Study, which was begun by sociologists at the University of Wisconsin, Madison, in 1957. The study enrolled one-third of that year's

Wisconsin high school graduates, with the intention of following them for decades in order to track their work experience, socioeconomic status, family life, trauma, and health. The participants came to my laboratory in the Brogden Psychology Building, a nondescript structure built in the mid-1960s in the center of campus whose most notable feature is the total absence of windows in the third-floor research wing. (The idea was that glimpses of the outside world would interfere with the serious experiments that were to occur there, but it's not obvious how making people feel as if they are inside a sarcophagus improves scientific productivity.)

Daren greeted each participant, explained the experiment and our reason for doing it, and had everyone sign a consent form (a requirement in all human research). We wanted to measure the brain's electrical activity, he said, to determine if people with greater left prefrontal activation were more resilient than those with greater right prefrontal activation. Then we carefully fitted a hairnet with electrodes sewn in place over each volunteer's scalp, first soaking each sensor's sponge tip in salt water so it would conduct electrical impulses better. From the control room next door, another assistant monitored the electrical contacts, yelling over the intercom when one needed to be fixed: "Eighty-seven in the right frontal region; thirty-six in the right parietal region!" (In that case, we would use a syringe to drip a little more salt solution onto the electrode's sponge.) Each participant got a plastic cape to keep the drips off his or her clothes, so between the electrode-studded hairnets and the capes it looked like we were running a futuristic beauty salon.

Once the sensors were recording properly, we measured baseline brain activity for eight minutes, four with the eyes closed and four with them open. Then we presented fifty-one pictures on a video monitor, each for six seconds. One-third of the pictures depicted upsetting images such as a baby with a tumor growing out of its eye; one-third showed something happier, such as a radiant mother embracing her infant; one-third showed a neutral scene such as a nondescript room. Sometimes during or after a picture, the volunteer would hear a short burst of white noise that sounded like a click—the "startle probe"—which tends to make people blink involuntarily, as described in the previous chapter. Finally, we placed sensors just below one eye over the orbicularis oculi muscle, which contracts when the eye blinks. A large body of previous research had established that when people are in a negative emotional state, their startle-induced blinks are stronger than during a neutral emotional state, while a positive emotional state tends to reduce the strength of a startle-induced blink compared with a neutral state. These sensors would tell us the strength of the blink, thus letting us track emotional state, both when people saw emotional pictures and afterward. That way we could gauge how quickly they recovered from a negative emotion elicited by a disturbing picture.

What we found, in a nutshell, is that people with greater activation on the left side of the prefrontal cortex during the baseline period recovered much more quickly even from the strongest feelings of disgust, horror, anger, and fear evoked by the images. From this, we inferred that the left prefrontal sends inhibitory signals to the amygdala, instructing it to quiet down, as indicated in the diagram below. This inference jibed with research from other labs, which found that people with *less* activation in certain zones of the prefrontal cortex show *more* long-lasting amygdala activity in the wake of an experience that evokes a negative emotion; they are less able to turn off negative emotion once it is turned on. Our research found essentially the flip side of that: Activity in the left prefrontal cortex *shortens* the period of amygdala activation, allowing the brain to bounce back from an upsetting experience.

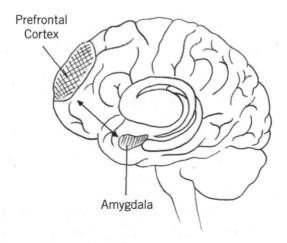

Resilience: Signals from the prefrontal cortex to the amygdala, and from the amygdala to the prefrontal cortex, determine how quickly the brain will recover from an upsetting experience.

Fast-forward to 2012. Thanks to MRI we now know that the more white matter (axons that connect one neuron to another) lying between the prefrontal cortex and the amygdala, the more resilient you are. The less white matter—the fewer the highways leading from the prefrontal to the amygdala—the less resilient.

Let me quickly add that this is the kind of statement that makes people think, *Oh great, I must not have many connections between my prefrontal cortex and amygdala, so I'm doomed to melt into a neurotic puddle every time I experience adversity.* As I'll explain in chapter 8, we now know that the brain is fully able to increase connections between regions, and in chapter 11 I'll explain how you can do so for these particular prefrontal-to-amygdala connections. Similarly, it is eminently possible to raise your baseline level of activity in the left prefrontal cortex.

To summarize the two extremes of the Resilience continuum: People who are Slow to Recover, having great difficulty bouncing back from adversity, have fewer signals traveling from the prefrontal cortex to the amygdala. This can arise from low activity in the prefrontal cortex itself or from a paucity of connections between the left prefrontal and the amygdala. Those who are Fast to Recover from adversity and are thus extremely resilient show strong activation of the left prefrontal cortex in response to setbacks and have strong connections between the prefrontal cortex and the amygdala. By damping down the amygdala, the prefrontal cortex is able to quiet signals associated with negative emotions, enabling the brain to plan and act effectively without being distracted by negative emotion—not a bad working definition of Resilience.

The Socially Intuitive Brain

I can thank Timothy, who was a high-functioning autistic boy of thirteen when I met him as part of a study, for helping me grasp that Social Intuition is a key dimension of Emotional Style, one whose extremes of Socially Intuitive and Puzzled reflect clear differences in brain activity and connectivity. Timothy was very intelligent and able to understand language and speak. His speech was quite monotonic, however, lacking the modulations called intonation contours—the stresses and changes in pitch, tone, and pacing that convey emotion. For example, when volume and pitch both increase, you can be pretty sure that your interlocutor is angry. When pace slows, volume decreases, and pitch flattens, the speaker is likely sad. Timothy's voice sounded like a robot's.

Even more striking, however, was his failure to make eye contact with whomever he was speaking to. He would make occasional fleeting glances toward me as I spoke with him, but most of the time his eyes focused elsewhere, anywhere but on mine. When we brought Timothy into the laboratory, eye-tracking software confirmed it: When we displayed pictures of faces on a video monitor, he spent very little time looking at the eye region, something that typically developing children fixate on. And when we put Timothy in the MRI tube and examined the patterns of activation in his brain as he looked at pictures of faces with neutral or emotional expressions, he showed much lower levels of activation in the fusiform face area, which specializes in deciphering faces, compared with typical children. And the less activation Timothy showed in the fusiform, the worse he did when we asked him to tell us what emotion a face was conveying. During this task Timothy also showed heightened activation in the amygdala. But when he averted his gaze from the eye region of a face, the level of amygdala activation fell. Timothy had implicitly learned a strategy to help him reduce the discomfort and anxiety he felt when looking into people's eyes.

We Homo sapiens are highly visual creatures, gathering social signals from our fellow humans with our eyes. From studies of children, adolescents, and adults like Timothy, I concluded that the lack of social intuition and the resulting failure to grasp what is socially appropriate comes from low levels of activation in the fusiform and high levels of activation in the amygdala, as shown in the diagram below:

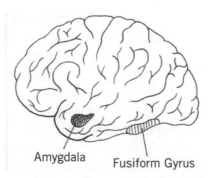

Amygdala   Fusiform Gyrus

Social Intuition: Low levels of activity in the fusiform and high levels in the amygdala characterize the Puzzled extreme of this dimension, while high activity in the fusiform and low to moderate levels in the amygdala are marks of a Socially Intuitive brain.

This is the characteristic brain pattern of someone who falls at the Puzzled end of the Social Intuition dimension. In contrast, someone with high levels of fusiform activation and low-to-moderate amygdala activity is Socially Intuitive, highly attuned to social signals and able to pick up even subtle cues.

Since we published this account of the autistic brain in 2005, a number of studies from other laboratories have confirmed that activity in the amygdala accounts for some of the variation found in people's social sensitivity. Several experiments, for instance, have focused on a molecule that reduces activation in the amygdala. Called oxytocin, this hormone burst into the popular imagination in the 1990s with research on little mammals called voles. Prairie voles are among the few species of mammal that practice until-death-do-us-part monogamy; a related species, the montane vole, adheres to the more common one-night-stand style of relationship. The main reason for the difference in behavior between the two kinds of vole, which are at least 99 percent identical at the genetic level, is that prairie voles are awash with oxytocin during key moments in their relationships—or the vole equivalent thereof—whereas montane voles are not. Moreover, the faithful and romantically committed prairie vole has abundant oxytocin receptors in its brain, while the feckless and unattached montane vole does not. In people, too, oxytocin has been linked to maternal behavior (it is released during childbirth and breast-feeding), romantic attachment, and feelings of calm and contentment.

Of course, human behavior is too complicated to boil down to levels of a brain hormone; for one thing, there is good evidence that feelings of love and attachment can themselves raise levels of oxytocin, rather than (or possibly in addition to) vice versa. But in any case, experiments with oxytocin have confirmed the role of the amygdala in the social brain: When oxytocin was spritzed into the noses of study volunteers, which allows it to go directly to the brain, it reduced activation in the amygdala. This suggests that quieting of the amygdala is the mechanism by which oxytocin induces feelings of commitment and attachment, and that quieting the amygdala by other means accomplishes the same ends—including laying the groundwork for a Socially Intuitive brain.

The Context-Sensitive Brain

The six dimensions of Emotional Style emerged, as I have said, serendipitously, in the course of my research on emotions. In the case of the Sensitivity to Context dimension, the monkeys did it.

In 1995 I began collaborating with my friend and colleague Ned Kalin on a study of the neural bases of anxious temperament in rhesus monkeys. To conduct the study, we obviously needed a way to identify such a temperament—to determine which monkeys were neurotic messes and which were well-adjusted, mellow bundles of fur. Ned started with the well-known fact that both human toddlers and monkeys tend to freeze when they encounter an unfamiliar situation, a form of anxiety called behavioral inhibition, and designed a study in which he exposed rhesus monkeys to the profile of a human. Monkeys who see a human silhouette, even on a video monitor, usually freeze. How long they stay frozen, however, is highly variable from one monkey to another, ranging from about ten seconds to longer than a minute.

Out of a hundred monkeys shown human profiles, we identified fifteen who stayed frozen much longer than the others. Curiously, three of the fifteen also froze from time to time when they were alone and not exposed to people. So not only did these three monkeys show an extreme response to a situation in which it is normal to show some response—that is, seeing a human profile—but they also showed an extreme response to a situation that does not trigger any response among most monkeys, namely, just sitting around their familiar home in the monkey colony with nary a human in sight. That was a clue that the monkeys were unaware of context: They confounded a safe, familiar situation with a novel and potentially threatening one, responding to the familiar as if it were unfamiliar and thus threatening.

The ability to distinguish a familiar from an unfamiliar context comes from the hippocampus, shown in the diagram on the following page.

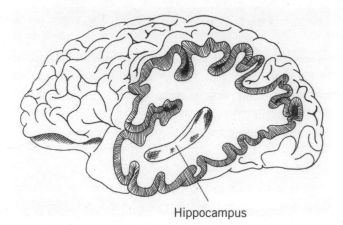

Hippocampus

Context: Although better known for its role in forming long-term memories, the hippo-campus also attunes behavior to particular contexts. Low activity is characteristic of the Tuned Out extreme, higher activity of being Tuned In.

The hippocampus is better known for its role in processing memories: It seems to act as a holding pen for short-term memories, getting some of them ready for transfer to long-term storage. But in a recent study of rhesus monkeys with Kalin, we found that the anterior hippocampus, the portion closest to the amygdala, is also involved in regulating behavioral inhibition in response to different contexts.

This discovery jibes with the discovery that people suffering from post-traumatic stress disorder often have abnormal hippocampal function. You prob-ably know of PTSD as the crippling condition in which normal experiences trigger painful memories of a past trauma, such as the sound of a car backfiring causing a war veteran to think he is again patrolling the violent streets of post-invasion Tikrit. But you can also think of PTSD as, more fundamentally, a dis-order of disrupted context: The anxiety and even terror that people with PTSD feel is quite appropriate in certain contexts, such as a battleground, but the prob-lem is that they experience these feelings in nontraumatic contexts. Experienc-ing a surge of adrenaline and amygdala activity when you hear an explosion as a marine marching into a war zone is expected and even adaptive; reacting that way to a *boom!* from a construction site in your neighborhood is not.

This was driven home to me in 2010 when I launched a study exploring whether meditation and other forms of mental training developed by the contemplative traditions can reduce some of the distress felt by war veterans. As I explained the proposed research to the commander of returning troops in Wisconsin, he told me what had happened to one of his soldiers that very week. Having just returned home from Afghanistan, the veteran purchased the motorcycle he had long dreamed of. He took his wife for a ride. When an ambulance raced by with sirens blasting, the vet panicked. Gunning the engine, he took off like a bat out of hell, lost control, and crashed. He was instantly killed; his wife was critically injured. It was a tragic demonstration of what can happen when the brain fails to grasp context—in this case, distinguishing between the significance of a sudden loud noise heard in the relative safety of the bucolic countryside and the significance of one heard in a war zone.

Numerous studies have found that PTSD is associated with a loss of volume in the hippocampus. That makes sense: A diminished hippocampus would have trouble forming memories of the context in which something traumatic occurred, conflating the dangers on the streets of Afghanistan with the safety of those in Wisconsin. From that, I've concluded that unusually low activity in the hippocampus underlies the Tuned Out end of the Sensitivity to Context dimension. At the Tuned In extreme, hyperactivity in the hippocampus is likely to cause an excessive focus on context, which can inhibit emotional spontaneity. This happens when someone who is hyper-focused on social context becomes emotionally paralyzed, so intent on parsing every nuance of the social environment that—like a dinner guest taking her place at an elaborately set table and finding six forks flanking her plate—she is afraid of making the wrong move. Similarly, someone who is extremely sensitive to context might shape her behavior to what she thinks the situation demands, presenting herself as one kind of person to her spouse, another kind to her boss, and still another kind to her friends, until soon she begins to doubt her own sincerity and authenticity.

Differences in the strength of the connections between the hippocampus and other brain regions, particularly the prefrontal cortex, underlie differences in Sensitivity to Context. The hippocampus communicates regularly with the brain's executive-function areas in the prefrontal cortex as well as sites of long-term memory storage, elsewhere in the cortex. Stronger connections from the hippocampus to these regions increase sensitivity to context, while weaker connections underlie insensitivity to context.

There is now an abundance of research, in both people and lab animals, implicating the hippocampus and the structures with which it communicates in encoding information about context as well as retrieving that information from storage. In studies of lab rats, for instance, "context" is as rudimentary as the flooring material of a cage or the size of the cage. To test rats' understanding of context, researchers pair a neutral stimulus, such as a tone, with an unpleasant one, such as a mild electric shock, which causes the rat to scurry around the cage in an attempt to get away from the zap. If every time the rat hears the tone it gets a little shock, it quickly comes to associate the tone with the shock, with the result that it starts scrambling as soon as it hears the tone, not waiting for the actual shock. (This experimental paradigm goes all the way back to Pavlov, who paired a tone with food in experiments with dogs. After enough experience of "tone equals food," his dogs began salivating in anticipation of the food after just hearing the tone.) But if the tone is then presented over and over without the shock, the rat learns that the shock is not a prelude to pain and stops scrambling when it hears the tone—a phenomenon known as extinction learning. Here is where context comes in: If the rat learns to stop pairing the tone with the shock while living in a small cage with a wire floor, when it is moved to a large cage with a solid floor it goes back to believing that tone equals shock and behaving accordingly. But the rat can manage this only if its hippocampus is intact. If the hippocampus is damaged, the rat will no longer distinguish between the two contexts and will instead fail to display extinction learning in either. Findings such as these strongly suggest that the hippocampus is important for context learning. Since learning presupposes perception, it makes sense to conclude that activity in the hippocampus underlies the perception of context.

The Self-Aware Brain

Back in graduate school, I began to study a personality type characterized by what was then called repressive defensiveness. People with this personality deny experiencing much anxiety or stress, yet their bodies tell a very different story, as we saw in one particular experiment. We had participants do what's called an emotional-phrase association task, in which they would say the first words that came into their minds when they read a phrase. The phrases were neutral ("The lamp is on the bedside table."), sexual ("The prostitute slept with the student"), or aggressive ("His roommate kicked him in the stomach"). The subjects who had high levels of repressive defensiveness rated the emotional phrases as not perturbing them at all—yet their heart rate and skin conductance (which measures sweating and hence anxiety) were off the charts. Clearly, these were not the most self-aware people. Subsequent research showed that people with marked repressive defensiveness do not consciously suppress their reactions, or lie about not feeling them. Rather, they are honestly oblivious to what is happening inside them. As a result of the failure to accurately perceive their internal states, what they say about how they feel diverges wildly from objective measures of those states.

At the time, there wasn't much more I could learn about this extreme lack of self-awareness, but that changed with the advent of neuroimaging. A key region of the brain for self-awareness is the insula, shown in the diagram below:

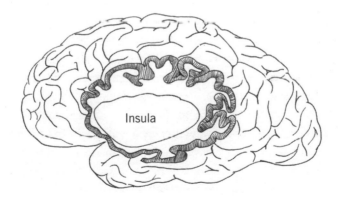

Self-Awareness: The insula receives signals from the visceral organs, with the result that high levels of activity support high levels of Self-Awareness and lower activity marks low levels of Self-Awareness.

Located between the temporal and the frontal lobes, the insula contains what is called a viscerotopic map of the body. That means the visceral organs—

heart, liver, colon, sexual organs, lungs, stomach, kidneys—are each mapped to a specific spot within the insula. By "mapped," I mean something akin to how each spot on the skin is mapped on the somatosensory cortex, where distinct clusters of neurons receive signals from every spot on the surface of the body, from our forehead to our toes and every sensitive spot in between. Each region of the skin sends signals to only one spot in the somatosensory cortex; in this sense, the surface of the body is *mapped* onto the somatosensory cortex. The insula similarly receives signals from our visceral organs and forms a map of them in the sense that specific regions of the insula receive input from specific organs. It is therefore the brain's monitoring station for everything below the neck and within the body. The insula also sends signals to the organs, instructing the heart to beat more quickly, for instance, or the lungs to inhale more rapidly. In addition to the insula, recent research shows, the somatosensory cortex is also involved in perceiving internal sensations. Next time you are aware of your heart racing when you feel scared or your face reddening when you're furious, you can thank both your insula and your somatosensory cortex.

Not surprisingly, then, the insula snaps to attention when it receives instructions (from other areas of the brain) to monitor heart rate. When this structure dials up its activity—by bringing online more neurons that receive input from the heart, for instance, or by enlisting more neurons to transmit these data to regions in the brain that do the actual counting—people are more sensitive to their heart rate. British researchers have found through neuroimaging that people who are more accurate in estimating their heart rate also have a larger insula; the larger the insula, the better the estimate.

Interestingly, higher insula activation is associated with greater awareness not only of physical sensations but also of emotions. In a 2010 study, also in Britain, scientists had people answer questions designed to assess where they fall on a scale of alexithymia (difficulty identifying and describing one's feelings). They indicated whether various statements accurately described them, such as: "When other people are hurt or upset, I have difficulty imagining what they are feeling"; "When asked which emotion I'm feeling, I frequently don't know the answer"; "I can't identify feelings that I vaguely sense are going on inside of me." Later, they measured the participants' insula activity. The more alexithymic someone seems from answers to such questions, the lower the insula activity.

What this all adds up to is that individuals with high levels of Self-Awareness have greater activation in the insula, while those with low levels of Self-Awareness have decreased activation. In the extreme, ultrahigh levels of insula activity seem to be associated with the excessive awareness of bodily cues that sometimes occurs in, for instance, panic disorder and hypochondrias. People with these illnesses are hypersensitive to their pulse, respiration rate, temperature, and other measures of anxiety and tend to overestimate them. As a result, a slight uptick in, say, heart rate that someone else might pay glancing attention to, perhaps wondering if something just beneath conscious awareness triggered a stress reaction, is interpreted as a sign of an impending heart attack.

The Outlook Brain

The 1982 discovery that greater activity in the left prefrontal cortex underlies positive emotions, while greater activity in the right prefrontal cortex is associated with negative emotions, was only the opening bell in the quest for the brain basis of what would become the Outlook component of Emotional Style. This early discovery was based on EEG—sensors applied to the scalp that detect the electrical echoes of brain function. While this was the only tool available for the study of the intact human brain for quite some time, once functional magnetic resonance imaging (fMRI) was developed, around 1995, it quickly became the method of choice to study brain function. In addition to having better spatial resolution than EEG, fMRI measures activity not just at the cortical surface, as EEG does, but also in subcortical regions such as the amygdala, which EEG cannot reach. (Just to be clear, fMRI uses the same equipment as standard MRI, used to look for tumors in the abdomen or bleeding in the brain, starting with the tube or tunnel that contains the powerful magnets. The "functional" part comes from the software that takes raw data about blood oxygenation changes in the brain and turns it into the striking pictures that have become ubiquitous.)

In 2007, I sat down with Aaron Heller, a terrifically talented graduate student who had joined my lab in 2005, to figure out a way to identify the specific aspects of positive emotion that are lacking in people suffering from depression. That might seem ridiculously obvious—depressed people aren't happy, right?—but in fact depression is marked by the absence of other positive emotions, too. Depressed people have little drive to accomplish goals, for instance (if they were lab rats, we would call this a lack of approach behavior), and sometimes they do not notice, let alone perk up, when they encounter something novel, the way other people notice a new batch of flowers in a neighbor's garden or a new coffee bar that just opened down the street. They also tend to lack persistence. Many depressed people are perfectly aware that they have plans (even if someone else made them, such as for a family outing) and to-do lists, but they seem to lack the tenacity required to carry them out. It is as if their drive gets short-circuited. Aaron and I wanted to identify the brain basis for these tendencies.

As we planned how to go about this, I remembered a study I had done fifteen years before and never published. I had shown depressed patients film clips chosen to induce positive emotions such as happiness, including scenes from a Steve Martin movie. Depressed patients reported as much positive emotion in response to these clips as nondepressed participants, challenging the notion that people with depression are unable to experience joy or other positive emotion. If there was a difference in how depressed people experience positive emotion, it wasn't reflected in how they responded to these comic film clips. But this study did not test for what I suspected would be a key difference between depressed and healthy people: how well they can sustain positive emotion, as opposed to how much they can feel.

To test this idea, we advertised for volunteers in local newspapers and on the local weather channel (a very good place to find depressed patients who are always on the alert for threats in the environment, something that the weather channel, particularly in Madison, often highlights). We wound up with twenty-seven people suffering from clinical depression and nineteen healthy volunteers. Since we wanted to measure brain activity while people looked at emotionally evocative pictures, we rigged up a system that let us project images onto the ceiling of an MRI tube.

When the volunteers arrived at my lab at the Waisman Center, they were escorted to a room with a mock MRI scanner, so they could see how they felt in the tube (this acclimates them to the procedure and lets anyone who feels too anxious either to bow out or try to get it under control enough to participate). Since the real MRI scanner sounds like a jackhammer two feet from your head, we digitized the sounds of the real scanner and blasted them into the mock one so people would know what they were in for. If they were going to freak out, it was much better that they do it in the mock scanner and not waste valuable scanner time.

Those who were still willing to participate then slid into the real MRI tube, headfirst on their backs. Once they told us they felt comfortable (everyone had headphones so they could hear us in the control room and a microphone so they could speak to us), we started projecting pictures onto a screen above their faces. All the pictures depicted something joyous, or at least something designed to bring a faint smile to the lips—children playing and clearly enjoying themselves, adults dancing, people eating food that looked good enough to make a mere observer salivate.

For each image, the volunteers got one of two instructions: either to simply view the pictures as they normally would, with no attempt to modify their emotional response, or to try to enhance and sustain the positive emotion the picture induced for as long as possible (or up to twenty seconds) after the image vanished from the screen. Some cognitive strategies they might try for prolonging the emotion, Aaron told them, were to think of themselves in the happy situation shown in the picture, or to imagine that the individuals shown were close family members or beloved friends, or to imagine that the joy they felt would last and last. Such strategies, we suspected, would intensify and possibly extend the initial happiness that people feel in response to seeing the images. All told, we showed the volunteers seventy-two images over the forty-five minutes they spent in the MRI tube. Aaron and I sat in the control room, where we monitored the protocol and ensured that the computers presenting the pictures and collecting the fMRI data were all functioning correctly. We also monitored the brain images to ensure that the participants were lying still. (If they move a lot, the images on the monitor get jumpy.)

From the data on all the volunteers, depressed and healthy, a clear pattern emerged. When the volunteers first saw the pictures depicting happy situations, activation in what we think of as the brain's reward circuit—marked in the illustration on the next page—shot up. This circuit is centered on a region in the ventral striatum, which is located below the cortical surface in the middle of the brain and has been shown in other studies to become active when people anticipate receiving something rewarding or pleasurable. More specifically, what becomes active during such experiences is a cluster of neurons within the ventral striatum called the nucleus accumbens, a region critical for motivation and generating a sense of reward. (It also happens to be packed with neurons that either release or capture the neurotransmitter dopamine, which plays a role in positive emotion, motivation, and desire; and endogenous opiates, which provide the famous runner's high.) Levels of activity in the nucleus accumbens were pretty much the same in depressed and nondepressed volunteers looking at the smile-inducing pictures. Everyone was able to feel an initial uptick of sympathetic joy. But that similarity did not last. Healthy people were able to maintain an emotional high for the entire session, but in depressed patients the positive feelings evaporated within minutes.

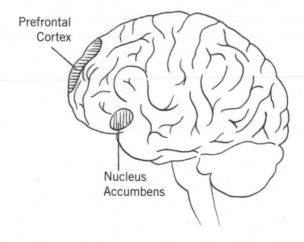

Outlook: The prefrontal cortex and the nucleus accumbens in the ventral striatum form the reward circuit. Signals from the prefrontal maintain high levels of activity in the ventral striatum, a region critical for generating a sense of reward, and thus a Positive Outlook. Low activity in the ventral striatum, due to less input from the prefrontal cortex, is a mark of Negative Outlook.

Why? The reason is that the nucleus accumbens receives signals from the prefrontal cortex, the higher-order region that transmits the instruction to intensify and maintain the happy feeling. This suggests that it is possible to think yourself—I'd go so far as to say *will* yourself—into feeling rewarded. Persistent signals from the prefrontal cortex basically tell the nucleus accumbens, "Don't let up yet! No flagging!" This is what happened in the brains of the healthy volunteers—but not in the brains of those suffering from depression. As time went by, in depressed patients the barrage of "Keep it up!" signals from the prefrontal cortex to the nucleus accumbens declined, and as a result activation in the reward-processing circuit did, too. It seemed that the messages were either not being transmitted from the prefrontal cortex or were being lost en route, like water dribbling out of a leaky hose.

We wanted to see what the decline in activity in the reward-processing circuit meant for real-world behavior, so after their session in the MRI tube we had the volunteers fill out a simple questionnaire. It listed different positive emotions such as happy, interested, inspired, and proud, and asked them to rate on a five-point scale how well the adjectives described their current mood. The ability to sustain activation in the reward-processing circuit strongly predicted the intensity of positive emotion people reported. The better people were at sustaining the neural glow from seeing a picture of children playing, the happier they reported feeling. Importantly, this was true of both the depressed patients and the healthy controls. On average, people with depression were deficient not in inducing but in sustaining activation in the reward circuitry and prefrontal cortex.

Recent findings in laboratory rodents suggest that the dopamine activity in the nucleus accumbens may be associated with the motivational component of reward, which underlies drive and persistence, while the endogenous opiates in the nucleus accumbens may be more associated with feelings of pleasure. When the opiate receptors in the nucleus accumbens are activated, they stimulate an adjacent brain region, the ventral pallidum, which, according to animal studies, may directly encode hedonic pleasure.

These findings indicate that activity in the nucleus accumbens and prefrontal cortex underlies the ability to sustain positive emotion. The greater the activity in the nucleus accumbens—activity sustained by signals from the prefrontal cortex—the further toward the Positive end of the Outlook dimension someone falls. Lower activity in this region underlies a Negative outlook.

The Attentive Brain

We swim in a sea of constant stimuli. It is nothing short of miraculous that we can focus attention at all, given the profusion of information that enters our brain every moment, to say nothing of the countless thoughts that pop into consciousness. Our ability to focus even some of the time is a monumental triumph of attention, allowing us to select some external or internal objects for conscious awareness and ignore the rest.

Humans have the capacity to focus attention through two related mechanisms. One is to enhance the strength of the signals in the attended channel; that is, we can increase the strength of the visual signals carrying the image of the characters we are reading relative to the strength of the visual signals carrying the images of, say, our hands holding this book. The second mechanism is to inhibit the signals in the ignored channels. We often use both strategies. Just think of the last time you were in a noisy restaurant, engaged in conversation with a companion. In order to hear him, you turned up the internal volume of his voice while simultaneously inhibiting sounds from surrounding tables. Even infants have a capacity for selective attention, being able to focus on their mothers' faces and ignore distractions from other sensory sources.

Two forms of attention are relevant to Emotional Style: selective attention and open, nonjudgmental awareness. Selective attention, as I explained in chapter 3, refers to the conscious decision to selectively focus on certain features of one's environment and ignore others. This capacity is a key building block for other dimensions of Emotional Style, since the failure to selectively attend can make it impossible to be Self-Aware or Tuned In. Open, nonjudgmental awareness reflects the ability to take in signals from the external environment as well as the thoughts and feelings popping up within our brain, to broaden our attention and sensitively pick up on the often subtle cues that continuously impinge upon us—but to do so without getting stuck on any one stimulus to the detriment of the others.

As long ago as graduate school I suspected that individual differences in selective attention were fundamental to emotional differences (this was before I developed the model of Emotional Style). Back then, I did a study in which I administered a questionnaire developed by psychologist Auke Tellegen, of the

University of Minnesota, which is designed to measure your propensity to become so absorbed in activities that you become unaware of your surroundings. (The student who is so focused on her math test that she doesn't hear the fire alarm? High on the Tellegen scale.) It asks people to rate how accurately various statements describe them, such as "I can be greatly moved by eloquent or poetic language," "While watching a movie, a TV show, or a play, I may become so involved that I forget about myself and my surroundings and experience the story as if it were real and I were taking part in it," and "When I listen to music I can get so caught up in it that I don't notice anything else."

After giving the Tellegen questionnaire to 150 Harvard undergraduates, whom you'd expect to be a highly focused bunch, we selected the top ten and the bottom ten scorers on absorption—in the scheme of Emotional Style, those with a Focused Attention style and those with an Unfocused style. We took EEG measurements from these twenty extremists as we presented visual and tactile stimuli (flashing lights and soft taps on the forearm from a device I rigged up). We instructed them to count the lights or the taps and recorded activity in their visual and somatosensory cortices as they did.

You might not expect that how lost someone gets in music is related to how strongly his brain responds to flashing lights, but there you are: How active the visual cortex became when a participant counted lights and how active the somatosensory cortex became when he counted taps were correlated with scores on the Tellegen Absorption Scale. People who are able to become completely absorbed in their surroundings showed stronger selective attention— more activity in the visual or somatosensory cortex during the relevant activity—than did those who do not get even slightly absorbed. This was my first clue that attentional differences might be important.

It was only by using modern brain-recording techniques, however, that I was able to identify the brain circuitry that controls where someone falls on the Attention dimension of Emotional Style. Other studies had already shown that the prefrontal cortex plays an important role in guiding selective attention; it actually boosts signals it wants to attend to (such as the words of our restaurant companion relative to the background chatter) and attenuates signals it wants to ignore (the other conversations). With this as our guide, we did an experiment in which we fitted participants with headphones and piped high- and low-pitched tones into them, one per second to either the right ear or the left. Participants were asked to press a button each time one type of tone was presented to one particular ear—the high-pitched tone in the left ear during one five-minute period, say, then the low-pitched tone in the right ear for the next batch, and so on for each of the four permutations. At the same time, we measured brain electrical activity with a dense array of EEG sensors all over the scalp.

Using modern methods of analyzing brain electrical signals, we found something quite striking. The more participants were able to steadily focus their attention on the correct stimulus, and so press the button only when a low pitch sounded in the right ear (for instance), the more the electrical signals from the prefrontal regions were synchronized precisely with the arrival of the tones. This "phase-locking" means that brain activity can be entrained to external stimuli; when it is, attention becomes highly focused and stable, as evidenced by the accuracy of the button presses and the consistency in the participants' response times from one trial to the next. The phase-locking that we identified involved only signals from the prefrontal region, not other brain regions, underscoring the importance of the prefrontal cortex in the regulation of selective attention.

Open, nonjudgmental awareness also arises from specific patterns of brain activity, as we discovered in a 2007 study of attentional blink. As described in chapter 3, attentional blink occurs when your mind, still dealing with a previous object of attention, becomes briefly unaware of your environment. It is not that you drop into a coma but that you are inattentive to what is happening right in front of you—such as a number popping up in a stream of letters. When we measure brain function during the attentional blink task, we find that the extent to which people overfocus on the first number (the 3 in T, J, H, 3, I, P, 9, M . . .) determines whether they will notice the second number (9). Or, put another way, people with a high degree of open, nonjudgmental awareness tend to notice the second number, while people with a low degree almost always miss it. The EEG data revealed the brain basis for this: the appearance of an event-related potential called P300. An event-related potential is simply an electrical signal that is elicited in response to a specific external event or stimulus; P300 refers to a positive (hence the P) response that occurs approximately 300 milliseconds following an event. Too strong a P300 signal indicates too much investment in focusing on the first number, which makes you miss the second; too weak a P300 indicates too little investment, which makes you miss the *first* number as well. The quality of open, nonjudgmental awareness implies a balance, so you do not get stuck on an engaging stimulus but are, instead, open to all stimuli.

To sum up: At the Focused extreme of the Attention dimension, the prefrontal cortex exhibits strong phase-locking in response to external stimuli as well as moderate activation of the P300 signal. At the Unfocused extreme, the prefrontal cortex shows little phase-locking and an extremely weak or extremely strong P300 signal.

I've thrown a lot of brain findings at you in this chapter, but I hope you have come away with two clear messages. The first is that there is an unmistakable pattern of neuronal activity underlying each dimension of Emotional Style. The second is that this activity often occurs in regions of the brain that would have astonished research psychologists in the 1970s and even 1900s. As I described in chapter 2, they didn't think much of emotions, assuming they were little more than annoying flotsam that got in the way of the brain's more august functions, namely, cognition, reason, judgment, and planning.

In fact, the circuitry of the emotional brain often overlaps with that of the rational, thinking brain—and I think there is a strong message in that: Emotion works with cognition in an integrated and seamless way to enable us to navigate the world of relationships, work, and spiritual growth. When positive emotion energizes us, we are better able to concentrate, to figure out the social networks at a new job or new school, to broaden our thinking so we can creatively integrate diverse information, and to sustain our interest in a task so we can persevere. In these cases emotion is neither interrupting nor disrupting, as the 1970s view held; it is facilitating. A *feeling* permeates virtually everything we do. No wonder, then, that circuits in the brain that control and regulate emotions overlap with those involved in functions we think of as purely cognitive. There is no clear, distinct dividing line between emotion and other mental processes; they blur into each other. As a result, virtually all brain regions play a role in or are affected by emotion, even down to the visual and auditory cortices.

These facts about the neural organization of emotion have important implications for understanding why our perceptions and thoughts are altered when we experience emotions. They also help to explain how we can use our cognitive machinery to intentionally regulate and transform our emotions, as we will soon see. But they raised a question. The brain signatures of each dimension of Emotional Style seem so fundamental to our being, it's easy to assume they are innate, as characteristic of a person as his fingerprints or eye color, and equally unlikely to change. At least, I made that assumption, as I'll describe in the next chapter.

CHAPTER 5

■ ■ ■

How Emotional Style Develops

When I first discovered the neurobiological bases for the six dimensions of Emotional Style, I assumed they were innate and fixed, established as soon as a child enters the world. Like other scientists (and new parents; our daughter, Amelie, was born in 1981, and our son, Seth, in 1987), I noticed and marveled at the striking personalities newborns have—something that comes into really stark relief if you have more than one child. Some infants are curious and laid-back; others are fussy and anxious. Amelie was a sunny, outgoing child who spoke early and took to it with gusto: She provided a running commentary on the world from her stroller, and by the time she was eight, she preferred to sit apart from my wife and me on airplanes. By the end of the flight, she had the life history of her seatmate. Seth, in contrast, was sweet and engaging but more apt to test the waters rather than dive right in.

Emotional DNA

Children, in short, seem to come into the world with preexisting temperaments and Emotional Styles, suggesting that they must be shaped by the genes they inherit from their parents. After all, a newborn has not had any life experiences that could influence her Emotional Style, which leaves only genes as presumptive determining factors.* And indeed, studies comparing identical twins with fraternal ones have produced compelling evidence that genes push us to be shy or bold, risk-taking or cautious, happy or unhappy, anxious or mellow, focused or scattered. These studies start from the fact that identical twins arise from a single fertilized egg and thus have identical gene sequences—those ribbons of chemical "letters" designated A, T, C, and G that spell out what the gene does (or, more precisely, what protein the gene codes for). Fraternal twins come from two different eggs fertilized by two different sperm and thus have the same degree of genetic relatedness as non-twin siblings, sharing roughly half the genes that come in different forms. (Many human genes come in only a single variety, so no matter how two people are related, they have identical copies of such genes.) Identical twins are thus twice as similar genetically as non-twin siblings and should thus be about twice as similar as fraternal twins on any traits that have a genetic component. Put another way, when the similarity between identical twins is greater than it is between fraternal twins for a particular trait, that's a strong sign that the trait has a genetic basis.

Twin studies have therefore been a gold mine for clues to the genetic basis of temperament, personality, and Emotional Style. Among the traits that are more similar in identical twins than in fraternal, and thus have a strong genetic basis, are shyness, sociability, emotionality, tendency to experience distress, adaptability, impulsivity, and the balance of positive and negative emotions. While this may seem like an odd assortment, I have chosen these traits because they each reflect one of the dimensions of Emotional Style:

- Shyness and sociability are related to where you fall on the Social Intuition dimension.
- Emotionality is related to Resilience and Outlook.
- A tendency to become distressed is related to Resilience.
- Adaptability primarily reflects Sensitivity to Context.

---

*New studies show that the intrauterine environment has an effect on physical health, including the likelihood that a child will grow up to develop heart disease or other adult illnesses. It may well have an effect on emotions, personality, and temperament, but if so, that has yet to be shown.

- Impulsivity is related to where you fall on the Attention dimension (being Unfocused tends to make you more impulsive).
- Generally positive or negative emotions are products of the Resilience and Outlook dimensions.

For all of these, the genetic contribution varies from 20 percent to 60 percent; that is, the difference between one person and another on these traits ranges from about one-fifth to three-fifths. Whether that seems high or low to you depends on your perspective. A strong genetic determinist would regard anything below 100 percent as suspiciously low, while someone who believes we enter the world as a blank slate would see even 20 percent as improbably high. To give you some benchmarks, the heritability of sickle-cell disease is 100 percent, while the heritability of belonging to a specific religion is close to zero.

Although living in this age of genetics has made many people assume that every trait is a product of our inherited DNA, that is clearly not so. Take schizophrenia. Although the disease has a strong genetic component, when one identical twin develops the disease there is only a fifty-fifty chance that the other will (identical twins are therefore said to be 50 percent "concordant" for schizophrenia). Depression has an even more modest genetic contribution and one that seems to vary by sex: In women the heritability of depression is about 40 percent, while in men it is about 30 percent. Interestingly, how easily a baby can be soothed seems to have little to no genetic component, and my own studies of twins show that anxiety disorders have even a smaller genetic component than depression. Even in traits with some genetic component, genes are not everything. Genetic propensities can aim a child down a path that leads to a particular Emotional Style, but certain experiences and environments can move the child off that path and onto another.

Born Shy?

The pioneer in the study of the innate basis for temperament has been Jerry Kagan, of Harvard, whom I got to know during my first year at grad school. A consummate scientist, Kagan was (and is) passionate about his research on how a child's temperament develops. Whenever I or my fellow grad students would pass him in the halls of the psych building, he would impishly ask, "Has nature lifted her veil for you today?" as he pushed and prodded us to discover what determines how a child turns out. Those were the days when you could smoke in your office, and Jerry's pipe gave his office an unmistakable olfactory signature.

Kagan pioneered the study of behavioral inhibition, which is basically a form of anxiety. The term describes the propensity to freeze in response to something novel or unfamiliar, as discussed in the context of the monkey studies in chapter 4. In everyday terms, it looks a lot like shyness. Kagan was the first scientist to systematically examine the behavioral and biological correlates of individual differences among young children with this quality of temperament.

His major finding came from a years-long study of scores of children who had been assessed for behavioral inhibition when they were young and classified as either behaviorally inhibited or uninhibited, and then assessed again in their early twenties. Kagan had parents describe their children and rate them on a scale of behavioral inhibition, observed the children himself, and also performed fMRIs of their brains. The latter showed that young adults who were categorized as strongly inhibited as toddlers showed heightened activation of the amygdala compared with those who were uninhibited as toddlers. The amygdala plays a key role in fear and anxiety, responding to threatening events in the environment. Heightened activation in the amygdala reflects an important characteristic of behaviorally inhibited children as well as adults: They are hypervigilant, constantly on the lookout for potential threats and sources of danger. They are likely to startle in response to small noises that most other people find innocuous. The bottom line of Kagan's work: Behavioral inhibition is a remarkably stable feature of temperament. The shy nine-year-old becomes the shy sixteen-year-old becomes the shy adult. Since Kagan had found what seemed to be the brain basis for that—heightened amygdala activity—and since at the time period of this work (the 1980s and 1990s) most scientists believed that inherited genes shape brain structure and function, the immutability of behavioral inhibition became part of popular culture. A typical headline: "Born Shy, Always Shy."

Until a few years ago, saying there is a genetic basis for Emotional

Style—or indeed for any other trait, physical or psychological—implied something else: that the trait would be with us for life, a legacy we would carry to the grave. After all, the genetically based shape of our nose and color of our eyes don't change (barring trauma or the ministrations of a cosmetic surgeon). Neither, went the conventional wisdom, would genetically based psychological traits such as Emotional Style.

But then a revolution swept through genetics, and the dogma that "genetic equals unchangeable" was toppled as thoroughly and dramatically as the statue of Saddam Hussein in Baghdad. Scientists made two startling, and related, discoveries: that a genetic trait will be expressed or not depending on the environment in which a child grows up, and that the actual gene—the double helix that winds through every single one of our cells—can be turned on or off depending on the experiences we have. It is popular to say that no single factor, genetic or experiential, accounts for variations in Emotional Style. But that's as obvious and uncontroversial as saying the sun is kind of hot. Something much more interesting is happening. Contrary to the popular belief that if something is genetically based we're stuck with it for life—for how can we change our very DNA?—even genetically based traits can be dramatically modified by how parents, teachers, and caregivers treat children and by the experiences children have.

Nurture's Effect on Nature

The reason genetically based traits can be altered is that the mere presence of a gene is not sufficient for the trait for which it codes to be expressed. A gene must also be turned on, and studies of both people and lab animals have shown that life experiences can turn genes on or off. In the terms of the shopworn debate called nature vs. nurture, nurture is able to act on nature.

That became clear from studies of a gene that became notorious in the late 1980s, when scientists began studying an extended Dutch family that included fourteen men who had committed impulsive, aggressive crimes including arson and attempted rape. In 1993, scientists reported that all fourteen had the identical form of a gene on the X chromosome. The gene makes an enzyme called MAOA, or monoamine oxidase A, an enzyme that metabolizes neurotransmitters such as serotonin, norepinephrine, and dopamine. The normal, or long, version of the gene produces lots of MAOA; the aberrant, or short, form produces low amounts. The more MAOA enzyme in the brain, the faster these neurotransmitters are broken down.

About one-third of people have the short form of the MAOA gene, while two-thirds have the long form. Studies in animals had linked low MAOA levels, typical of the short form of the gene, to aggression, perhaps because when MAOA is in short supply the brain remains jacked up on neurochemicals in a way that induces aggression. Indeed, men with the short form of the MAOA gene tend to have a hair-trigger response to threat, as measured by a surge in activity in the brain's fear region—the amygdala—at the sight of an angry face. That might explain the violence committed by the men in that Dutch family. The MAOA gene became known as the "violence gene," headlines warned of "violence in the blood," and there was talk of screening everyone to identify carriers of the short form, the better to thwart budding criminals before they were even old enough to walk.

But then came a remarkable study. Scientists determined the MAOA status—benign long form or notorious short form of the gene—of 442 males in New Zealand. The scientists then pored over criminal and other public records to determine which of them had exhibited antisocial or criminal behavior by age twenty-six, conducted a psychological assessment to ascertain whether each had antisocial personality disorder or adolescent conduct disorder or other psychological illness, and interviewed at least one person who knew him well. Sixty-three percent of the men had the high-activity form of the MAOA gene, and 37 percent had the low-activity form. Here was the surprise: There was no statistically significant association between MAOA gene status and antisocial behavior. That is, sometimes low-activity-MAOA boys grew up to be criminals or delinquents, and sometimes they didn't. But the "sometimes" was eye-opening. If a man with the low-activity MAOA gene had been abused as a child, as 8 percent had been, he was extremely likely to exhibit antisocial behavior. Those with the exact same gene who had been loved and cared for, which described 64 percent of the men in the study, had no greater risk of antisocial behavior than high-activity-MAOA males. Genes alone did not increase the risk of delinquency and criminality; that required a bad environment, too.

The scientists followed up this study by looking at the same New Zealanders to see whether a similar nature-nurture dance was going on with another gene that had been linked to behavior, namely, the serotonin transporter gene. This gene, located on chromosome 17, makes an enzyme that whisks serotonin, a neurotransmitter, out of synapses. It thus has essentially the opposite effect of the popular antidepressants called SSRIs (selective serotonin reuptake inhibitors), which keep serotonin in synapses longer. Not surprisingly, a short version of the gene, which results in less serotonin transporter being produced, has been linked to depression. But again the scientists showed that genes are not destiny. Of men with the short version of the transporter gene, only those who had suffered stressful life events in their early twenties had a high risk of depression. Having the "depression gene" but a basically trauma-free life meant no greater risk of depression.

These were the first hints that our emotional and psychological fate does not lie solely within the twists of the double helix. Depending on the experiences a child has had, a genetic basis for shyness, or aggression, or delinquency might or might not manifest itself. Rather than thinking of DNA as the software running our cells—or the player-piano sheets that dictate what notes will be played—it is time to think of it as a music collection. Whether you store your music on an iPod or as a stack of CDs or (are there any of us left?) vinyl records, what music we hear depends on which music gets played. Just because we have it doesn't mean the harmonies encoded in the bumps and valleys within the grooves of an LP will reach our ears. Now we know that just because we have a particular gene doesn't mean that its music will be part of our lives. Or, if I may abandon the music analogy, think of it this way: Genes load the gun, but only the environment can pull the trigger.

But how, exactly, might the life we lead reach into the very genes in our cells and turn them off or leave them on? As usual, the first hints of how DNA can be silenced or amplified by our experiences came from studies in lab animals. Back in the 1990s, biologist Michael Meaney began to wonder about some rats he was studying. Some were extremely anxious and inhibited; these were the little guys who froze when they were dumped in unfamiliar surroundings and jumped a foot in the air when startled. They were neurotic messes, leaping out of their skins in response to a stressful experience and releasing a flood of stress hormones called glucocorticoids, which get the heart pumping and the muscles primed for flight or fight. Other rats were laid-back and relaxed; placed in an open field they had never seen before, they explored as happily as teenage girls in a new shopping mall. They handled stress with aplomb: When given an electric shock, for instance, they released only a trickle of glucocorticoid stress hormones. Once mellow female rats became mothers, they regularly licked and groomed their pups, in the rodent version of hugging, kissing, and tucking them in at night with a bedtime story. Anxious rats, in contrast, were too neurotic to attend to their maternal duties. They were so derelict in licking and grooming that if there were a rat-world child protective service agency, it would make them attend parenting classes.

The reason some rats shrug off stressful experiences so nonchalantly, Meaney and his colleagues discovered in 1989, is that they produce fewer glucocorticoids in response to stress. Just as a child who is very sensitive to his mother's requests doesn't have to be asked twice to clean his room, so it is with rats that are very sensitive to glucocorticoids: A little bit of stress hormone goes a long way, so less of it floods their bodies in response to a stressful experience. With less stress hormone coursing through their blood, the rats seem more mellow, less jumpy, less fearful, less neurotic. And the reason some rats are more sensitive to stress hormones is that their brains contain more receptors for them, in the hippocampus. Receptors, as their name implies, serve as docking stations for glucocorticoids. With a profusion of receptors, the body doesn't need to produce as much stress hormone to get the message across— just as if your teenager had three ears, you wouldn't have to yell at him so loudly to stop leaving food-encrusted dishes around his room (perhaps).

In the mid-1990s Meaney discovered that the reason some rats had more glucocorticoid receptors in their brains, and hence tolerated stress better, was that their mothers lavished licks and grooming on them. This experience made a lifelong difference to the baby rats, programming their brains to shrug off stressful experiences and not turn them into quivering balls of hairy protoplasm when exposed to unfamiliar surroundings. Pups whose mothers had licked and groomed them grew up to be laid-back in response to stressful experiences, curious, eager to explore new surroundings, and resilient in the face of stress. But baby rats whose mothers rarely licked and groomed them grew up to be fearful and stressed out, hypersensitive to being startled and prone to freezing in fright at anything unfamiliar or unexpected.

Since neurotic, anxious female rats gave birth to neurotic, anxious baby rats, everyone assumed that anxiety and neuroticism were genetic, inherited, and—of course—fixed. And since laid-back female rats gave birth to laid-back baby rats, everyone assumed that mellowness was genetic, inherited, and fixed. But Meaney had long been skeptical of the dogma that anxiety or mellowness is inherited like eye color. He therefore opened a sort of rodent adoption agency, having neurotic mothers raise pups born to mellow mothers and mellow mothers raise pups born to neurotic ones. Nurture trumped nature. Pups born to anxious, neurotic, neglectful mothers but raised by attentive mothers grew up to be laid-back, frisky, curious, and all-around well adjusted (for rats), happy to explore unfamiliar terrain and taking new situations in stride—just like their adoptive mothers. Pups born to nurturing, mellow mothers but raised by neglectful mothers got the short end of the stick: Despite their promising genetics and start in life, they grew up to be little bewhiskered bundles of nerves, jumping out of their skin when startled and cowering in fear when thrown into an unfamiliar environment. And there was one more change. When the adopted rats grew up and became parents themselves, the females behaved like their adoptive mothers rather than their biological ones: Those born to neglectful mothers but raised by mothers that had dutifully licked and groomed them treated their own offspring the same, while females born to conscientious mothers but raised by neglectful ones also neglected their own offspring. The rats had inherited a *behavior*—from mothers whose genes they did not share. It was a triumph of nurture over nature.

You might conclude that the mother rats somehow taught their adopted offspring how to behave and how to treat their own offspring, or at minimum modeled anxious or mellow behavior for them. But Meaney thought something more profound might be at work. He knew that one of the genes that cause a rat to be anxious produces those receptors for stress hormones in the hippocampus—the ones that mellow rats have lots of and neurotic rats have few of. As you recall, the more receptors, the fewer stress hormones that are produced in response to, say, seeing a hungry feline off in the distance, and thus the fewer stress hormones that are available to make the brain a stressed-out, neurotic mess. Conversely, the fewer the receptors, the higher the production and availability of stress hormones, and the more anxious and neurotic the rat. An obvious place to look for an explanation of the baby rats' nurture-over-nature transformation, therefore, was these hormone-receptor genes.

What Meaney and his colleagues found was that the gene ordering up production of the stress-hormone receptors is altered by early life experiences: The gene is about twice as active in pups reared by an attentive, nurturing mother as in pups reared by a neglectful one. (Remember, the more active gene produces more glucocorticoid receptors. The more receptors, the mellower the rat.) The precise molecular mechanism by which this happens, Meaney discovered, is that a mother rat's licking and grooming allows the glucocorticoid-receptor gene to be turned on. But if a rat mother is neglectful, rarely licking and grooming her pups, the gene for the stress-hormone receptor is silenced: A cluster of atoms (called a methyl group) literally sits on the gene and shuts it off. Meaney had thus shown that life experiences can reach down into an animal's very DNA and amp it up or quiet it down. The result was so startling that one of the world's top science journals turned Meaney down when he submitted the paper for publication; the notion of the environment turning genes on or off decisively overturned too much dogma. (Meaney found more sympathetic editors at *Nature Neuroscience*, which published his study in 2004.)

People are not rats, but our DNA can also be silenced by methyl groups, as Meaney soon found in another groundbreaking study. He and his team availed themselves of a grim but precious scientific resource, the Quebec Suicide Brain Bank. As the name implies, the bank contains samples of brain tissue from people who have taken their own lives, all preserved in Pyrex containers in a freezer at the Douglas Mental Health Institute in Montreal and backed up with full psychological and medical histories. Meaney studied samples from thirty-six brains: one-third from suicides who had suffered abuse in childhood, one-third from suicides who had not been abused, and one-third from non-suicides. Analyzing the human brains as they did the rats', he and his colleagues found that, compared with non-suicide brains, the brains of people who had taken their own lives and had suffered child abuse contained significantly more methylation "off" switches on the gene for the glucocorticoid receptor. That was the gene Meaney's team had discovered was methylated in rats raised by neglectful mothers. In people, as in rodents, when this gene is silenced the stress-response system is on a hair trigger, making it extremely difficult to cope with life's adversity. Abnormal activity in the stress-response system had long been linked to suicide. With this 2009 discovery, Meaney had completed the causal chain: Child abuse alters the expression of genes in the brain, this altered expression impairs the ability to cope with adversity, and the inability to cope with adversity leaves the individual more vulnerable to suicide.

Contrary to the belief that the genes we carry are fixed and unchanging, studies like Meaney's are showing that our DNA is more like that extensive CD collection: Just because you have a CD doesn't mean that you will play it, and just because you have a gene doesn't mean that it is turned on (or, as geneticists say, "expressed"). Instead, the extent to which genes are expressed is strongly affected by the environment. Thus, while we may have, say, a genetic propensity for anxiety, being raised in an environment that nurtures equanimity can silence that "anxious DNA" and prevent it from having an effect in the brain and thus on our behavior or temperament. It is as if we never slip that CD into the player.

The presence of a methyl group sitting on a piece of DNA is called an epigenetic change. It does not alter the sequence of the gene, denoted by the well-known strings of A's, T's, C's, and G's, but it does alter whether that gene will be expressed. And it may explain puzzles like the low concordance for schizophrenia between identical twins. At birth, identical twins are very similar epigenetically; if a particular gene is silenced in one twin, it is usually silenced in the other. But as we go through life, it turns out, we accumulate epigenetic changes. Either through random chance or because of the experiences we have—something akin to being nurtured by a parent, perhaps, but almost certainly many others that reach down into our very DNA—our genes take on more and more epigenetic marks, silencing some genes that had previously spoken and lifting the gag order that others had been under.

A 2005 study showed how important experiences are for this: Identical twins who led similar lives and spent more of their lifetimes together were more similar epigenetically than identical twins who had different lifestyles and lived more of their lives apart, which presumably meant they shared fewer experiences. By age fifty, twins reared apart had four times as many epigenetic differences—four times as many genes that were silenced in one twin but not the other—as they had at age three, when their life experiences were close to identical. And that's the secret of how a different environment translates identical genomes into different people.

Enter Robie

I have often fantasized about measuring changes in gene expression in children as they grow older . . . especially after our Robie the Robot study. Our first major longitudinal study of Emotional Style, it analyzed behavioral inhibition, the trait that Kagan had famously found to persist from childhood into adulthood. Inhibition tracks the Resilience dimension of Emotional Style; that is, inhibited or shy children are less resilient. They take longer to recover from any situation that causes them to feel stress, such as being in an unfamiliar environment or having to interact with strangers. Uninhibited children tend to exhibit Resilience; they take such situations in stride, recovering so quickly from any initial frisson of anxiety that they barely notice it. Indeed, I would argue that this very lack of Resilience may in fact underlie and be more basic than shyness: Because speaking to strangers, exploring unfamiliar terrain, and otherwise acting in a bold, behaviorally uninhibited way causes shy people anxiety and distress that lingers for a long time, they avoid such situations. They act shy. (People who are Self-Aware consciously avoid such situations, while those who are Self-Opaque do so unconsciously; the latter say they just happen to prefer to work from home and to stay in every night.) Given my belief at the time that children have inborn Emotional Styles, and that those Styles persist throughout life, I assumed that we would find that a child's Resilience (or lack thereof) stays with her forever—fixed, stable, immutable.

In the 1980s our local newspaper carried birth announcements, a gold mine for scientists in need of study volunteers. An office here at the University of Wisconsin dutifully entered each birth, building up a vast database of children organized by birthday. If a scientist wanted, say, a few hundred three-year-olds, all she needed to do was request the list of children born three years earlier and start cold-calling parents. Which is what we did: We went down the list of children born in 1985 (this was 1988), eliminated any who lived more than twenty-five miles away, and asked the parents if they would be interested in participating in scientific research on behavioral inhibition—shyness. We got 70 percent to agree, a reflection of the esteem in which the university is held, and we began scheduling them to come to my lab.

Although we had a few fathers, mostly mothers brought their toddlers—368 of them, two families at a time. My graduate student Rona Finman escorted the mothers to chairs in a corner of a large playroom strewn with toys and asked them to fill out a pile of questionnaires asking for basic demographics as well as their child's temperament (moody? anxious? shy?) and their own. The children, meanwhile, played on the floor with the toys—blocks, dolls, trucks, and the like.

After a few minutes, the door to the playroom opened and in rolled a remote-control robot, Robie. Just a little shorter than the toddlers, he scooted along on three wheels, his eyes a pair of blinking lights, his head able to swivel left and right, and his mechanical mouth moving when he spoke. Rolling closer to each child under our remote-control commands, he announced in a computerlike voice, "Hi, I'm Robie the Robot, and I've come to play with you. Will you play with me?" The mothers, per Rona's instructions, remained focused on the questionnaires and did not look up or interact with their child.

The kids' reactions were all over the map. Some scampered up to Robie and touched and talked to him. Others sat frozen in place, not uttering a word. Will, for instance, the son of a teacher and an administrator in a state agency, was one of the frozen. As soon as Robie rolled in, Will dropped the toy he was playing with and stood stock-still, speechless and staring at the robot. He remained intensely vigilant, his face wary, watching Robie for the first sign of trouble. When the robot moved closer to him, Will backed up several steps and then resumed his frozen stance. After several additional invitations to play, Robie announced that he had to leave, turned around, and left through the door he'd come in. We could practically see Will exhale; he came alive and got back to playing. In contrast, Sam, the son of a small construction business owner and a librarian, ran right over to Robie as soon as the robot entered the room, smiling and grabbing him and talking nonstop. Rona was certain the kid would break off the antenna from Robie's head, which would have left us unable to control him with the remote joystick. Sam jumped up and down with Robie and called to his mom ("Look! Look at the robot, Mom!") as she valiantly followed our instructions to focus on the questionnaires no matter what happened.

Multiply Will and Sam by 184 and you'll understand what we observed over twenty-five minutes of watching toddlers interact (or not) with Robie. We had scores of Wills, shy, reticent, wary, and not at all resilient; they were unable to overcome their fear of a strange being and a strange situation. And we had scores of Sams, extremely outgoing, sociable, and resilient, able to absorb the shock of a talking robot and adapt to the odd situation. In the prevailing jargon, we had kids who showed almost no behavioral inhibition and kids who showed a high degree of behavioral inhibition—lots of Resilience and non-Resilience, respectively. And we had scores of kids in between. Six months after this behavioral assessment (that's how long it took to do all the Robie trials), we asked the families back to the lab so we could obtain the children's baseline EEG activity. A "baseline" EEG measures brain activity when someone is just resting rather than doing anything in particular—though of course we couldn't control whether the kids were daydreaming or silently humming the *Sesame Street* song.

That toddlers vary enormously in how shy or sociable they are is hardly stop-the-presses news. You can witness the same thing by hanging out at the local sandbox. We were after something else. As I said, the prevailing paradigm in developmental psychology was that temperament persists. That's what we wanted to test.

Based on how the three-year-olds reacted to Robie, we identified 70 out of the 368 to follow more intensively, making this a longitudinal study. We identified roughly equal numbers of the shyest children like Will, who had spoken just a couple of words to Robie and buried their heads in their mothers' laps; bold ones like Sam, who spent less than ten seconds with their mothers and instead made Robie their new best friend; and children in the middle, who scored around the mean for how long it took them to engage with Robie and how much they spoke with him. We asked their parents to bring them back to the lab when the children were seven, and again when they were nine.

Given Kagan's finding that temperament seems to be a fixed trait, I expected that the children who were shy with Robie when they were three would be shy when we tested them again, and that toddlers who were outgoing would similarly have remained that way. But even well-respected findings in science are just begging to be tested, and there were a couple of things about the Kagan studies that raised some red flags, especially for a colleague who would prove invaluable in the Robie the Robot studies, Maureen Rickman.

As an undergraduate, Maureen majored in neuroscience at Madison at a time—the early 1980s—when it wasn't even officially offered; we had only a graduate program. But Maureen convinced the powers that be to let her construct a neuroscience major, and she became hooked. She spent five years after graduation doing research on infants, especially the development of hearing, but as she said recently, "I really wanted to do something that mattered. I heard there was this guy doing research on real people, doing EEGs to locate brain function in particular regions, and asking what do the brains of anxious people look like." That guy was me, and I took Maureen on as a graduate student.

I explained to Maureen that, much as Kagan did, we were going to ask whether the behavioral inhibition a child showed at age three would persist into late childhood, and whether the brain activity patterns that underlie that trait would persist as well. By the time Maureen inherited a spot on the longitudinal study, we were on the third assessment; the children were nine years old. Before she so much as saw a kid, Maureen's first task was to reread Kagan's "once shy, forever shy" studies, the ones that found that behavioral inhibition in childhood persists into adolescence. More than the conclusion, which was well known, it was the convoluted details of methodology that Maureen focused on.

One afternoon she came to my office and asked if I had noticed something about those studies: One of Kagan's measures of children's shyness was parental ratings. You know, Maureen said, that might be a problem: Parents tend to think about their child in a way that becomes almost set in stone. This child is "the rambunctious one." This child is "the smart one." This child is "the shy one." What if the habit of pigeonholing their kids had blinded parents to the changes in temperament their child had undergone? What if having seen the shyness in their three-year-old, parents thought of the child as shy forever? Might this have skewed Kagan's findings? Parents' ratings of their child wasn't the only measure Kagan used, but it was one of them, so this might be a problem.

There was another methodological red flag. Digging deep into the details of Kagan's study, Maureen noticed that another way he classified kids was by the lengths of utterances before their ninth spontaneous one. If you're confused by that, so was Maureen. Counting the number of words in the first eight things the kids said in various lab situations, and equating lower numbers of words with shyness but verbosity with lack of behavioral inhibition, came out of left field. Is a child who says, "Who's that?" shier than one who says, "Mommy, Mommy, who is that man sitting there?" Shyness makes some people so anxious they prattle on endlessly; it makes other clam up, Maureen argued. "How did he come up with this measure of shyness?" she asked me. "Whatever measure you choose has to have face validity and make sense, or else you need a really good explanation for why you did it that way."

Kagan also used more understandable measures of shyness: whether a child froze in the presence of a stranger, and how high his levels of stress hormones were in this encounter. But the two odd aspects of his methodology—parental evaluations and the number of words in a child's utterances—got us thinking that the conclusion about the persistence of shyness might not be as solid as everyone assumed.

Poof! Goes Temperament

Robie wasn't going to work with kids this old; for all we knew, nine-year-olds were as likely to deck the thing as to engage it. To test these children's behavioral inhibition, we therefore decided to place each of them in three different situations. In the first, we planted a stranger—one of my graduate students—in the room and had him sit reading a book as the child came in. Some of the kids immediately bounded over and asked, "What are you reading?!" while others ignored him and began playing with the toys. In the second situation, a scientist wearing a snarly wolf mask spoke to the child, then removed the mask and invited the child to touch and wear it. Some of the kids recoiled in terror, while others were eager to play. Finally, we ushered the kids into a room filled with slightly threatening playthings, such as a seven-foot-long tunnel, a balance beam, and a gorilla mask on a stand. We measured it all: whether and how soon the child approached the stranger on her own, whether she agreed to let the stranger sit by her on the floor and play, how many minutes before the child spoke to the stranger, how long it took for her to get within three feet of the stranger, how the child reacted to the wolf mask, and whether she played with the stuff in the "risk room."

In addition to observing the children's behavior, we made two additional measurements. As we had with the three-year-olds, we obtained baseline EEGs for the nine-year-olds six months later. At both ages, the bold children (those who had less behavioral inhibition, in the terminology of the experiment) had greater left than right activity in their prefrontal cortex, whereas the shy (more behaviorally inhibited) children had greater right than left activity.

I had seen this pattern of asymmetric frontal activity many times before: in people suffering from depression (greater right than left activity), in contented babies (greater left than right activity), in people watching amusing videos (greater left than right activity), and in people watching upsetting videos (greater right than left activity). But this was the first time the asymmetry was linked to anything that was not clearly an emotion. This time, we saw left-right asymmetry in conjunction with being bold or shy. At each age, we found high correlations between brain activity and behavior. Children with greater left- rather than right-side prefrontal activity were less inhibited, while those with the greatest right-side prefrontal activity had the most extreme levels of behavioral inhibition. Bold children recover quickly from setbacks and are able to get on with what they were doing without getting derailed by them. Shy children, on the other hand, have a much more prolonged response to adversity; that's why they freeze for long periods of time in unfamiliar situations. This confirmed my hunch that the Resilience dimension of Emotional Style is reflected in patterns of left-right asymmetry in the prefrontal cortex.

It took a full year to collect the behavioral and EEG data on each group of children and then another year to analyze it. Over the long months when the numbers were being crunched, we kept wondering whether the children's toddler selves would match their nine-year-old selves in terms of behavioral inhibition. When Maureen brought me the data, she could barely contain her astonishment. She had scrutinized each measurement—time to speak to the robot or the stranger, time to get close to the robot or the stranger, how many menacing toys a child played with—to calculate the correlation between its value when the children were toddlers and when they were seven and nine. Her astonishment reflected what she found, or, more accurately, what she didn't find: The correlation between the measures at age three, age seven, and age nine was nonexistent. Or, to be precise, the average correlation for the overall measure of behavioral inhibition from age three to nine was .03. For the non-statisticians among you, a correlation of 1 means that two quantities change in lockstep; your height in inches and your height in centimeters has a correlation of 1. A correlation of 0 means two quantities have no relationship to one another; the correlation between the number of wins the Yankees rack up in a given baseball season and the number of brides named Vera that year is 0.

The fact that the correlation between behavioral inhibition at age three and behavioral inhibition at age nine was .03 means only one thing: Behavioral inhibition is not a stable, enduring trait. "We have absolutely random re-sorting of the three groups—the shy, medium, and bold kids!" Maureen blurted out. "About one-third of the children in each group stayed in the group they started in, but look at all these others who moved around." Fully two-thirds of the children in each of the three initial groups (at age three) were in a different group at age nine.

We were taken aback by this contradiction of Kagan's conclusion, so I asked Maureen to consult one of the university's leading experts in child de-velopment and a statistics whiz, Hill Goldsmith, to be sure we weren't doing something wrong. Perhaps we had erred in how we combined measures such as how long it took a child to play with Robie, or to speak to the stranger, and everything else we used to classify children as shy or bold or in the middle. Based on what Hill told her, Maureen redid all the analysis—then showed up in my office again and said, with equal parts conviction and surprise, "They're still randomly distributed!" A child who was shy as a toddler had the same odds of being shy at age nine as she did of being bold or of being smack-dab in the middle. Ditto for bold toddlers, whose temperament a decade later could be predicted as accurately by flipping a coin as by knowing what he had been like at age three.

To be sure that there wasn't something squishy about our behavioral test, we also analyzed the children's patterns of prefrontal EEG activity. Maybe we had somehow messed up in our behavioral data, which are seldom unassail-able, but EEGs are completely objective. Yet this measure, too, torpedoed the dogma that temperament is fixed. In some children the EEG pattern at age three matched that at age nine, just as in some children behavioral inhibition persisted. But overall, the correlation between EEG pattern at age three and that at age nine was less than 0.1. And we were relieved to see that children whose pattern of brain function persisted over the years were also those whose behavioral inhibition remained about the same—another check on the validity of our measurements. The EEGs, showing relatively greater left or right prefrontal activity in bold or shy children, respectively, matched the behavioral data, in that kids with greater left activation were also the ones who befriended Robie and chatted up the stranger.

This was not what I had expected. Measures of brain and behavior at age three did *not* predict what the kids were like at age nine. For the majority, who they were at three—and what their brain was at three—was very different from who they were at nine. This was the first challenge to my own assumptions about the stability of traits that have a genetic basis, and it spurred my thinking about the plasticity of the human brain.

What was so compelling about the data was that, until then, the prevailing model of child development had been that if you're born at the far end of the spectrum for shyness and anxiety (these are the babies who shriek when someone clears his throat and cry inconsolably afterward), you become an anxious child and are at risk of developing an anxiety disorder. The model further held that if you are an off-the-chart bold child, you will climb furniture and sled down a staircase on a dinner tray, enjoying numerous trips to the emergency room as a result, and grow up to be a wild and crazy adolescent (and, as an adult, probably either a derivatives trader or a drug dealer). "But when you looked at our data, there was more change than stability in our kids' temperament," Maureen reminisced with me recently. "It wasn't that as they grew up they had more social skills, and so were able to engage with a stranger better while deep down still being an anxious kid. That's what the old model said: that people can slap an overlay of learning or socialization on their basic temperament, but that innate shyness or boldness would still be there. But we found that *the brain changed*. Once-shy kids were now in the middle or even in the bold group, and once-bold kids moved to the middle or even into the shy extreme. For two-thirds of the kids, the whole system—brain, physiology, temperament, and behavior—changed. This challenged the idea that temperament is highly stable.

"What we showed is that if you teach a child to speak when someone speaks to him, the underlying physiology changes and a shy kid can become a bold kid," Maureen continued. "If you expose your shy child to anxious situations—nothing extreme, more like putting her in the sandbox at the playground with other kids—and support her in those situations, you're teaching her to cope. With bold kids, you teach them to read the danger signals in their environment. You get them to stop and see what other children are doing, see that they don't always have to be the first in line or accept every dare. What we found in this study was change all the way down to their startle reactions. It wasn't just an overlay. It's not right to think of kids who were once shy as forever being, deep down, 'really shy,' even if they have stopped acting shy. We showed that you can change the 'deep down'; you can change the brain patterns that underlie shyness and extreme boldness."

Maureen left academia in order to practice child psychology here in Madison, but our groundbreaking discovery remains with her. "When I look at how this discovery informs my practice—I work with children from three years old up—I see that it has made me try to help people understand that there are individual differences, and that an individual difference doesn't have to be a problem. Maybe you're wired really tight, and noises make you jump. You have high sensory sensitivity associated with a nervous style. But the only time that style is a problem is when it's causing you problems. You don't have to think of these differences as pathologies. It's a *kind* of a kid, not a broken child. A lot of the parents who bring their child to me are incredibly relieved when I tell them they don't have to medicate their kid; they have to understand and advocate for their kid."

And the Meek Shall Inherit . . . Boldness

For an inkling of how and why a bold toddler can become a shy adolescent, and a shy toddler a bold adolescent, let's look at what happened with Will and Sam. Will, our fear-frozen toddler, had an outgoing younger sister and also was lucky to have teachers who nurtured his sociability. While he did not become an extremely outgoing child by age nine, he moved squarely into the middle of the distribution. Sam's dad developed cancer, for which he was hospitalized twice, when Sam was five and seven. This adversity understandably took a toll on the family, which may have played a role in moving Sam from being one of the most outgoing and sociable in our sample to the large clump of children in the middle.

Although neither Will nor Sam moved from one extreme to the other, they each moved closer to the center from their respective extremes of behavioral inhibition and lack of inhibition. About half the children moved in the other direction, from the center toward one extreme or the other. And some children did move from one end of the spectrum to the other. At age three, Shawn was one of our least inhibited toddlers; he walked up to Robie almost immediately, babbled to him nonstop, and smiled radiantly. I think he would have liked to drag Robie home to be his best friend. But when Shawn was eight, his father unexpectedly died of cancer. When we saw Shawn at nine, he was a changed child: He froze in the presence of strangers and wouldn't play with a single thing in the risk room. He had become one of the most inhibited children in our study.

Now you see why I would love to measure gene expression in people: It would be fascinating to know what happened to "shyness genes" in kids who cowered in the presence of Robie the Robot when they were toddlers but gleefully played with the masked stranger when they were in fourth grade. And I would love to know what happened to the shyness genes in kids who walked right up to Robie when they were three but shrank into a corner as nine-year-olds rather than engage the stranger reading in a nearby chair. I would love to know how living with a life-of-the-party sister affected Will's DNA, how every encouraging interaction with supportive teachers reached in and silenced some genes but turned on others. I would love to know how the high stress-hormone levels Shawn experienced seeing his father hooked up to tubes and wires in the hospital, the emotional shock he suffered at his father's death, and the anxiety he felt in the weeks and months afterward ("What will happen to me without my dad?") changed his very DNA. Unfortunately, although we know precisely where to sample for Meaney's stress-hormone-receptor genes in the brains of rats, in humans we don't. And even if we did, people tend to take a dim view of having tissue samples scooped out of their brains. A study like this can be done only in people who have donated their brains to research; Meaney's analysis of the brains of suicide victims is the best example.

This study of children was an early lesson for me in the power of brain plasticity. During development, some of the brain's most characteristic features, such as pattern of EEG activity in the frontal cortex, can undergo radical change.

How do we reconcile our discovery that there is essentially no stability in the trait of behavioral inhibition, at least from age three to nine, with Kagan's findings that there is? We subsequently realized that the extent to which a temperamental characteristic such as behavioral inhibition is stable over time is itself a stable individual difference. That is, in some people this trait persists from toddlerhood into early adolescence, while in others it does not. Thus, there appears to be a subgroup of children in whom behavioral inhibition and some of its associated brain-activity patterns are stable over time, while another subgroup in whom they are not. Kagan may have unintentionally studied only the first subgroup—kids in whom shyness persists through adolescence. But that is only about 15 percent of children. As we saw with Will, Sam, and Shawn, new environmental circumstances (supportive teachers, an influential sibling) and wrenching life experiences (the illness or death of someone close to you) can modulate temperament and Emotional Style. If our environment remains stable (and by "environment" I mean the kind of personal experiences we have, too), so will our temperament and Emotional Style. If it does not, Emotional Style will change.

These discoveries about the malleability of a key facet of Emotional Style—and indeed, of personality, temperament, and other genetically based traits—provide the foundation for parents and teachers to identify a child's Emotional Style and try to shape it. Even if a child has a genotype that predisposes him to be anxious, being raised in a relaxed and nurturing environment can dial down those genes, quite literally, by altering the extent to which particular genes are expressed. Similarly, a child who has a genetic predisposition for shyness can develop into a sociable adolescent and adult if her parents do not shelter her and indulge her shyness but instead gently encourage her to interact with other kids. The environment does not just shape behavior or even brain function. It also affects whether genes turn on or off and, therefore, which inherited traits we express.

CHAPTER 6

■ ■ ■

The Mind-Brain-Body Connection, or How Emotional Style Influences Health

Fingernails screeching across a blackboard. A stiletto stabbing your eyeball and being pushed in deeper and deeper. The blade of a knife being drawn slowly across the bottom of your foot. Wait, was that a footstep behind you?

I don't mean to give you the creeps. Well, actually I do, but for a reason: I want you to have a physiological reaction to something that is entirely within your mind. Maybe you don't wince and cover your ears at the sound (or thought) of fingernails on a blackboard, and maybe the thought and mental image of a sharp object impaling your eyeball doesn't send uncomfortable tingles radiating out from your seat the way it does mine. But I'm pretty sure there is *something* that you see or imagine that triggers a physiological reaction below the neck. Feelings and thoughts, which originate in the brain, literally get out of that gray matter and into the rest of the body. Indeed, William James thought emotion was nothing *but* the perception of body events. Without going that far, modern neuroscience has shown that emotions do infuse not only the mind but also the body: Feeling anxious raises your blood pressure and makes your pulse race, and feeling content can strengthen your immune system, with the result that you do not succumb to infections and other contagious illnesses as often as someone who is chronically down in the dumps.

From what I have told you thus far, you know that Emotional Style affects how we feel about ourselves and those around us, how we behave, how susceptible we are to stress, our cognitive function, and our vulnerability to particular psychiatric disorders. But Emotional Style also affects physical health. It has physiological consequences that in turn have important downstream effects on the function of our respiratory, immune, cardiovascular, gastrointestinal, and endocrine system—in short, on health below the neck. In fact, I would go so far as to assert that of all the forms of human behavior and psychological states, the most powerful influence on our physical health is our emotional life.

The founders of psychosomatic medicine, the study of the relationship between psychosocial factors and illness, had this intuition centuries earlier. The world's first physicians—men such as the Greek anatomists Erasistratus in the third century BC, Galen (Marcus Aurelius's doctor) in the second century, and the Persian philosopher Avicenna in the tenth century—all used pulse rate to make inferences about "lovesickness," believing that unrequited love would leave a mark on the sufferer's physiology. In one famous story related by Plutarch, Erasistratus was called upon by King Seleucus of Greece to diagnose his adult son Antiochus, who was near death with an illness no other physician could identify. Erasistratus observed that whenever the young man was in the presence of Stratonice, the king's new (teenage) wife, "Sappho's symptoms became then all too apparent, such as a break in the voice, blushing and downcast eyes, sudden perspiration and irregularity of the pulse," recounted Plutarch. "He also became subject to swoons, doubts, fears and sudden pallor. From all these manifestations Erasistratus drew the conclusion that the king's son loved nobody but her, and that he was determined to die rather than show it." (A happy ending ensued when the generous king gave his new wife to his infatuated son; no word on how Stratonice felt about this.)

Behavioral Medicine

Psychosomatic medicine has also been called mind-body medicine, partly because the term *psychosomatic* took on a pejorative cast, implying that whatever symptoms a person was suffering from were all in his head. These days it is usually called behavioral medicine or health psychology. By whatever name, it has racked up some notable successes. Studies have found that social isolation tends to increase levels of cortisol and other stress hormones, to raise blood pressure, and to weaken the immune system, with the result that most people who live alone and lack a robust social network produce a weaker antibody response to flu vaccines. As I emphasized in chapter 1, however, findings such as this reflect an average response and ignore outliers. If one were to study only people who are comfortable keeping to themselves—research that has not, unfortunately, been done—I suspect one would find that social isolation has no adverse physiological consequences. To the contrary: Forcing an introvert to be sociable would likely bring on these harmful effects.

At the other end of the spectrum, being socially engaged is associated with a lower risk of developing coronary artery disease, with catching fewer colds and other infections, and with a longer life. Again, this is not universally true; being a social butterfly is a good way to expose yourself to every germ that passes through your zip code. And if you are forcing yourself to attend parties, office functions, business outings, and the like without truly enjoying them— but, to the contrary, finding them stressful—then the longevity and immune-system benefits are unlikely to follow.

Behavioral medicine has also shown that depression raises the risk of dying from coronary artery disease. You might be tempted to protest that sad, lonely people do self-destructive things like smoking or drinking too much, and that this is the reason they have shorter life expectancies and worse health. But these studies take that possibility into account and have ruled it out as the causative mechanism. What is found over and over again is that— again, on average—the emotional state itself predicts the health problems.

Given that emotions have physiological consequences, it follows that Emotional Style does too: The patterns of brain activity that underlie particular dimensions of Emotional Style are associated with physiological systems that play a role in health and illness. What is in your brain necessarily influences what is in the body. Moreover, the communication is bidirectional, so what is in the body influences what is in the brain.

These statements should not be terribly surprising. After all, emotions clearly affect the body, as anyone who has been nauseated by extreme stress, felt her energy level soar in response to intense happiness, or been rendered insomniac by a profound sadness can attest. But until quite recently, few studies measured the mental and the physical (that is, outside the brain—what's called peripheral biology) simultaneously, largely because specialized areas of scientific research can be extremely insular. Someone who studies emotions would no more deign to measure something about the lungs or immune system than a Rolex repairman would take a look at your furnace.

Another reason why the role of emotions in health has not gained more traction in medicine reflects a real and important gap in the science. Although behavioral medicine has amassed impressive evidence documenting the role of psychosocial factors in illness, it has fallen short when it comes to mechanistic analysis. What has been missing, that is, is a toe-bone-is-connected-to-the-foot-bone level of explanation that connects an event in the brain (and as far as we know, all emotions have some representation in the brain) with consequences in the body. For health psychology to be taken more seriously and incorporated into mainstream medical practice, it must undertake more brain-based analyses of *how* psychological and psychosocial factors "get under the skin" and influence peripheral biology in ways that impact health. In short, it has to stop being so brainless.

I think that is quite achievable. One of the key discoveries about the six dimensions of Emotional Style is that they are associated with specific neural circuits and with specific patterns of activity in those circuits, as described in chapter 4. That gives us a starting point: How does *this* pattern of activity in *these* regions of the brain travel out of the skull and into the body to produce changes that affect health? And how do events in the body feed back and influence the functioning of the brain circuits that underlie Emotional Style?

The fact that Emotional Style affects physical health opens up a whole new world of possibilities and takes mind-body medicine to another level. For it suggests that you can control your feelings and thoughts in a way that will be good for your physical health, and that all of us—individual physicians, the medical establishment, and potential patients alike—should take the mind more seriously when it comes to understanding the causes of disease and devising ways to both prevent and treat it.

Don't Be Sick, Be Happy?

For decades, when health psychologists talked about the effect of emotions on health, they were almost always referring to negative emotions: anger, hostility, depression, fear, and anxiety. To be sure, there are mountains of evidence showing that, on average, negative emotions weaken the immune system, raise the risk of heart disease, and the like, as I mentioned previously. In 2005, when two prominent health psychologists counted the studies of depression and health and the studies of happiness and health that had been done up until then, they found over twenty times more of the former than the latter. Only recently have health psychologists turned to the effect of positive emotions: happiness, joy, contentment, eagerness, excitement, enthusiasm, and the like. But once they did, a whole slew of associations turned up, with the result that one of the strongest and most consistent findings in behavioral medicine now is the relationship between positive emotions and health. But establishing that relationship was a struggle. The reason had to do with yet another obstacle that psychosomatic medicine has had to overcome, namely, finding a reliable way to assess people's moods.

This might seem straightforward. Ask someone how generally happy or satisfied he is with his life, and you'd think you'd get an answer you could take to the bank, or at least to the laboratory notebook. In fact, however, people are surprisingly bad at this kind of reporting. How do we know this? Because although assessing how happy you are with your life should yield approximately the same answer from one day to the next—after all, your family situation, career, health, and other components of our sense of well-being don't vary from day to day (barring sudden catastrophe or lottery success)—in fact, people's assessments swing wildly, depending on when you ask them. Remember, the question is not "How are you feeling right now? What mood are you in?" but "In general, how satisfied are you with your life overall?" If people are asked about their general level of well-being on rainy days, they report being less satisfied with their life than when they're asked on sunny days. If they're asked the question after a rotten commute home, they also describe having a lower sense of well-being than if they're asked in the middle of a triumphant day at work or school.

Since the question is meant to get at things that are not affected by the weather or a bad commute, such as satisfaction with your marriage, contentment with your career, and pride in your children, this is clearly a problem. In particular, it is a problem for studies that look for an association with overall well-being and measures of physical health. If the assessment of well-being is, for the reasons given above, so unreliable, then any connection with health will be obscured. Indeed, for decades research on the link between overall contentment or well-being and health produced inconsistent results, in part because of the problems in measuring happiness.

Fortunately, psychologist Daniel Kahneman figured out that you can't trust people to honestly and accurately tell you how satisfied or happy they are with their lives—not when the answer depends on whether it's raining. Kahneman shared the 2002 Nobel Prize in Economics for seminal discoveries about judgment and decision making and has also done groundbreaking research on the biases inherent in measures of subjective well-being and how we might circumvent them. What he and his colleagues discovered is that you get a more consistent and more accurate measure of people's overall life satisfaction if, instead of asking them the question directly, you ask them to report on their momentary experiences and then aggregate the answers to construct an assessment of general well-being. In practice, this means giving people a beeper, cell phone, or other device and texting or calling them at random times over the course of weeks or longer. Every time the person is contacted, she reports how she is feeling right in the moment. When aggregated over many samples, the result is an index of happiness or well-being that is considerably less influenced by minutiae like whether rubberneckers made you late for dinner with your kids.

Once scientists figured out the left side of the equation (happiness levels), so to speak, they could get on with the task of assessing the right side of the equation (health) and thus whether well-being has any effect on the body. Just to be clear, when I refer to happiness levels I mean something enduring, what psychologists call a trait, not a state—a person's typical emotional experience, not fleeting responses to events. The whole point of the methodology Kahneman developed was to capture emotional traits rather than emotional states. One other important point: The studies I'll describe all used what are called prospective designs, which means they measured emotional traits (as well as health) at the beginning of the research and then determined whether a given trait predicts changes in health over the study period. Because the emotional state was measured before any change in health, the change in health cannot have been the *cause* of the emotional trait—that is, getting sick cannot be the cause of depression, and avoiding the flu year after year cannot have been the cause of the strong sense of contentment. The depression or the contentment came first. That means we are on firmer ground when we attribute subsequent changes in health to that baseline emotional trait.

This is not so in a good deal of other research on mind-body connections to health. For instance, studies have linked positive emotions to lower rates of stroke among elderly people living at home, to lower rates of having to return to the hospital among people with coronary disease, and to a greater chance of conceiving and carrying a baby to term among women undergoing assisted fertilization. These studies, although intriguing and suggestive, did not rule out the possibility that negative emotional traits were actually a marker of subclinical disease. That is, they did not eliminate the possibility that worse health caused the negative emotions (cardiovascular disease causes you to feel ill, so you have more negative emotions, for instance, rather than you have negative emotions and therefore develop cardiovascular disease), and better health caused the positive emotions, especially such specific ones as feeling energetic, rather than vice versa.

You have probably read that positive emotions have also been linked to better disease outcomes—the "Think positive and you'll survive breast cancer [or other life-threatening disease]!" idea. The evidence for this is actually equivocal. Not a whole lot of studies have tested this idea, and in those that have, the results are a mixed bag. My reading of this research, shared by many of the leading lights in behavioral medicine, is that positive emotions seem to be beneficial for patients with diseases that have effective treatments and decent odds of long-term survival, such as Stage I breast cancer, coronary heart disease, and AIDS. But high levels of positive emotion may be detrimental in people with advanced diseases that have poor prognoses, such as metastatic melanoma or breast cancer and end-stage renal disease. One reason might be that a consistently positive outlook—"*I'll be fine!*"—causes patients to under-report symptoms, and thus not receive the care they require, or makes them fail to take prescribed drugs or undergo recommended screenings or treatments. Sometimes too much optimism can backfire on you.

Several recent studies make a persuasive case for the health benefits of positive emotions. In one, Andrew Steptoe and Michael Marmot, of University College London—two of the world's leading experts on the psychobiology of health and disease—collected health and well-being data from 116 men and 100 women. All 216 were middle-aged British civil servants between the ages of forty-five and fifty-nine. The scientists then analyzed whether there was any association between well-being, as assessed in the reliable way that Kahneman had developed, and three important biological markers: heart rate, cortisol levels, and plasma fibrinogen levels. (All 216 people were also part of the famous Whitehall studies of public health, so dozens of biological and medical measurements had already been collected.) A lower heart rate is generally associated with better cardiovascular health, which is why athletes often have a heart rate down in the range of forty- or even thirty-something beats per minute. Cortisol is a stress hormone that is secreted into the bloodstream by the adrenal glands, which sit just above the kidneys, in response to signals of fear or threat or anxiety from the brain; it helps the body deal with acute stress by mobilizing resources and inhibiting inflammation, which can arise from injury associated with stress. But when too much cortisol is released, or when it is released unnecessarily—that is, not in response to an actual and immediate threat but in response to chronic background anxiety—it can damage the brain and body, even killing brain neurons. Plasma fibrinogen is a molecule implicated in inflammation and coronary disease. Because its blood levels rise in stressful life circumstances, it is a general marker of inflammation and has been implicated in such illnesses as diabetes, cardiovascular disease, and asthma.

The participants who rated themselves as the least happy had cortisol levels that were, on average, 48 percent higher than those who rated themselves as the most happy. The least happy participants also had a hugely elevated plasma fibrinogen response to two stress-inducing tasks: the Stroop test, in which participants must name the color ink in which a word is printed (not difficult for the word *piano*, but a bit of a brain twister when *red* is written in green ink or *blue* in brown ink); and tracing a star seen in a mirror image. On top of all this, participants were told the average person can complete the task in a certain number of seconds, which was much faster than people actually do it, so the participants felt quite stressed. But physiologically, people handled the stress very differently. In the least happy group, the average fibrinogen increase was twelve times greater than in the happiest group.

These findings clearly indicate that happiness is related to biological markers that play an important role in health. Importantly, Steptoe and Marmot didn't just leave it at that. They recontacted their volunteers three years later to repeat the physiological measurements. They found that people who scored high in positive emotion still had lower levels of cortisol and fibrinogen, as well as lower heart rates. The initial finding was no one-trick pony.

The next step was to determine whether happiness actually influences physical health. In one of the most convincing studies of this, health psychologist Sheldon Cohen, of Carnegie Mellon University, had 334 volunteers aged eighteen to fifty-five rate their emotions once a day for three weeks, every time they got a phone call from the scientists (the Kahneman method of assessing happiness and well-being). In particular, the volunteers reported how well a list of nine positive and nine negative adjectives described them—happy, cheerful, calm, at ease, lively, and energetic, for instance, or sad, depressed, nervous, and hostile. After this three-week mood assessment, the participants went to Cohen's lab, where one of the scientists placed an eyedropper full of a solution that contained rhinovirus, the virus that causes the common cold, in their noses. For the next five days, the participants were quarantined, living in the lab and passing the time by reading, watching movies, listening to music, sleeping, and eating. The highlight of their day was when a scientist would examine them for signs of a cold and, if they had caught one, how severe it was. One measure of that severity was congestion, determined by how long it took for a dye sprayed into the nostrils to reach the back of the throat. Another was the weight of the volunteers' used tissues.

Cohen and his colleagues found that participants with the highest levels of positive emotions were nearly three times less likely to develop a cold than those who reported the least positive emotions. They also found that participants who had the largest number of social interactions, particularly positive ones, were the least likely to develop a cold. These links held up even when the scientists accounted for the volunteers' baseline immunity (that is, whether a volunteer had antibodies to the cold virus at the start of the experiment). Interestingly, people with the most positive emotions tended to report fewer and milder cold symptoms for any given severity of disease; that is, if two people had equally bad colds as measured by congestion and mucus production, the more contented person reported fewer and milder symptoms, while the sadder or grumpier person (with identical symptoms) reported that this was a truly awful cold. This injects a cautionary note into studies of positive emotions and health: If you just ask people about their health, those with the highest levels of positive emotion are more likely to paint a rosy picture even if, objectively, they are no better off than their depressed, grouchy, or chronically angry neighbor. That's why it's important to do studies that actually measure illness, as Cohen does, rather than ask people about their rheumatoid arthritis, fibromyalgia, or other aspects of health.

No single study can establish a scientific fact, and so it is with the connection between happiness and health. Although the Cohen study is, to my mind, one of the most rigorous to have looked for this link, other excellent studies have come to the same conclusion. One enterprising team got their hands on journal entries, letters, and other autobiographical writings made by a group of young nuns (their average age was twenty-two), members of the School Sisters of Notre Dame religious congregation. On September 22, 1930, the Mother Superior of the order, who lived in Milwaukee, had sent a letter to all the nuns she supervised requesting that each sister write an autobiography. Many of the writings survived. These are what scientists led by David Snowdon, of the University of Kentucky, analyzed, by coding every word in 180 autobiographies that reflected an emotional experience as positive, negative, or neutral. When the scientists calculated the frequency of words and sentences conveying positive emotion, they found that the more there were, the greater was the probability a nun was alive sixty years later. Significantly, the frequency of words and sentences conveying negative emotions was not associated with a greater risk of dying young—an important hint that it was the presence of positive emotions, not the absence of negative ones, that supported living to a ripe old age.

Another excellent study followed sixty-five- to ninety-nine-year-old Mexican Americans for two years. It found that those with higher levels of positive emotion at the start were only half as likely to die over the following two years as those with lower levels of positive emotion. The reason this 2000 study stands out is that the researchers controlled for a long list of diseases (heart problems, stroke, cancer, diabetes, and arthritis), as well as being overweight, smoking, drinking, and levels of negative emotions. Even when they controlled for the presence of such life-shortening illnesses and habits, the association—positive emotions, less risk of dying soon—held up.

Also impressive is a 2001 study that measured positive emotions in healthy seniors. It found that lower levels of positive emotions at the start of the study was associated with a higher likelihood of having a stroke at some point over the next six years, especially in men. Again, these scientists ruled out a host of other factors—age, income, education, marital status, obesity, blood pressure, smoking, history of heart attack, diabetes, negative emotions—as explaining the differential risk of stroke.

In a convincing 2008 review of seventy studies in both ill and healthy people, scientists concluded that positive psychological well-being or happiness was associated with reduced mortality in both normal and diseased samples. For example, psychological well-being was linked to reduced cardiovascular mortality in healthy people and to reduced death rates in patients with renal failure and HIV infection.

Together, these and other findings (for I have described only a few of the dozens of studies examining positive emotions and longevity or disease) make a persuasive case for a relationship between happiness and health. In a nutshell, happier people show better health outcomes on a wide variety of measures, from cortisol levels to the likelihood of catching a cold, and also live longer. But I do not mean to imply that the case is closed. To the contrary, these studies had significant gaps, such as not completely disentangling the effects of having positive emotions from *not* having negative emotions. Might what seem to be the benefits of positive emotion merely be the benefits of not having negative emotions, since studies galore link negative emotions to disease? This may seem like splitting hairs, but it's not, for a very practical reason. On our Outlook scale, if the absence of negative emotions is all you need for good health, then it's fine to be in the middle, away from the gloomy, Negative end of the dimension. But if the presence of positive emotions is what counts, then to improve health you would need to move yourself toward the Positive end of the scale.

One other caveat about the association between positive emotions and health: Although the British study finding that positive emotions are linked to lower levels of cortisol and fibrinogen was an important step in nailing down the mechanism by which positive emotions affect health, there are still a lot of unknowns about how that correlation works. For one thing, people who feel contented, energetic, optimistic, and the like tend to take better care of themselves, getting the proper amount of sleep and exercising. They also tend to have better, closer social ties, which has been linked to a lower risk for disease and premature death. Finally, as Cohen points out, doctors and other health-care providers may take better care of pleasant people, perhaps going the extra mile to get them into a clinical trial for their life-threatening disease, spending more time with them to persuade them to adopt healthier habits, and the like. On the other hand, there are quite plausible mechanisms by which a brain state—this thing we call emotion—might get into the rest of the body and thereby influence health below the neck.

It was against this background of studies showing that emotions are correlated with physical health that I began to wonder whether specific Emotional Styles might be as well. Let me mention a few of the ways that even one Emotional Style, the Positive version of the Outlook style, might affect health:

- Perhaps the most obvious way is by influencing behavior. This may be somewhat anticlimactic, since positive emotions would affect health only indirectly, but it's important. A sense of well-being, the experience of joy, and enduring happiness are associated with eating a more healthful diet, exercising regularly, and sleeping better. All of these enhance health and the ability to fight off disease and decline, both physical and mental.

- Positive emotions can also act more directly on physiology, dampening the cardiovascular system and the neuroendocrine or hormone system. In both cases, the link might be what's called the sympathetic nervous system, the largely unconscious part of our nervous system that controls, among other things, the fight-or-flight response to threats. If the activity of the sympathetic nervous system were dialed down, heart rate would decrease; that is generally regarded as a marker of good cardiovascular health. Blood pressure would also fall, reducing your risk of stroke. Quieting the neuroendocrine system would lower blood levels of epinephrine and norepinephrine, the fight-or-flight hormones.

• One powerful mechanism by which positive emotions could affect health is through immunity: They have been shown to increase levels of growth hormone and the hormones prolactin and oxytocin. The first two have the ability to bind to white blood cell receptors, which can prime these immune-system attack dogs to be more vigilant and effective in vanquishing infection, while oxytocin decreases blood pressure as well as the stress hormone cortisol.

• There might even be a more direct effect of positive emotions on the body. Some neurons in the brain, called sympathetic fibers, connect all the way to the thymus and lymph nodes, which are production factories for immune-system cells. Activating these neurons in the brain via positive emotions might therefore activate the thymus and lymph nodes, unleashing infection-fighting cells. Sympathetic fibers also release a slew of substances that bind to receptors on white blood cells, again priming them to attack invaders.

These diverse possibilities make it that much more critical to nail down the actual mechanisms by which Emotional Style influences health. Before I describe our findings on how Emotional Style affects physical health, let me illustrate the strong connections between the brain and body with a little experiment we did recently.

Botox and the Body-to-Brain Connection

The conventional wisdom holds that the brain issues commands to the rest of the body and does all the directing, with the body below the neck meekly awaiting orders and never talking back. But it's actually a two-way street: Communication between the mind and body is bidirectional, and not only at the simplistic level of feeling upset if you stub your toe or blissful when you are getting a massage. The brain, it turns out, uses feedback from the body in basic information processing. For that discovery, we can thank Botox.

Since 2002 this drug (derived from botulinum, a neurotoxin produced by the bacterium *Clostridium botulinum*) has been used cosmetically to reduce frown lines. Botox paralyzes the muscles temporarily, usually for weeks or months, with the result that frown lines disappear. We weren't interested in the disappearing lines so much as the paralyzed muscles. At least as far back as Charles Darwin, as I mentioned in chapter 2, scientists have suspected that making a facial expression of emotion can cause us to feel that emotion: Smile and you'll feel at least a little happier; drop the corners of your mouth and you'll feel a little blue; frown and you'll feel somewhat angry. Using this "facial feedback hypothesis" as our guiding principle, we put out the word to cosmetic surgery clinics around Madison that we were in the market for female volunteers who had already scheduled appointments for Botox treatments of the corrugator supercilii muscle between the eyebrows, better known as the frowning muscle, to erase glabellar (frown) lines. These women, we realized, were walking, talking experiments in how to manipulate the feedback from the body—specifically, in this case, the face—to the brain.

I teamed up with a Madison colleague, psychology professor Arthur Glenberg, and his graduate student David Havas. One of their areas of research is how language is processed and understood, in particular how we comprehend emotional language. For the study, we tested the forty-one women before and after their first Botox injection, measuring how long it took them to read sentences meant to trigger different emotions. For an anger-inducing sentence, for instance, we chose "The pushy telemarketer won't let you return to your dinner." For sad, we used "You open your e-mail in-box on your birthday to find no new e-mails." For happy, we tried "The water park is refreshing on the hot summer day." If making the corresponding facial expression indeed enables people to more quickly process and better understand the emotion, then we would expect the post-Botox women to stumble a bit when they read angry or sad sentences: The corrugator muscle squeezes the eyebrows together into a frown when we're angry and raises the inner eyebrows when we're sad. Botoxed women cannot make the facial expressions that signify anger or sadness. We therefore predicted that the time it took the women to read angry or sad sentences should increase following the Botox injection. But because the corrugator muscle doesn't help us smile, its paralysis should not affect whether the women could grin, so we predicted that the time it took them to read happy sentences should be unaffected.

And that is what we found. We measured reading time by having each woman press a button as soon as she finished a sentence. To be sure they had really read it, we asked them a question about what they had just read after every few sentences. After their corrugator muscle was paralyzed, it took the women, on average, essentially the same amount of time to read the happy sentences (1.3 seconds) as it had taken them before the injection—but 1.55 seconds to read the sad sentences and the angry ones. That is, it took about a quarter of a second longer to read the angry and sad expression after Botox compared with before Botox, whereas there was no difference for the happy sentences. In the world of cognitive psychology and reaction time measures, a quarter of a second is an eternity and was a highly significant difference. Blocking the activation of muscles involved in forming angry or sad facial expressions slowed reading times for sentences that convey and induce anger or sadness—emotions that normally activate the corrugator muscle. What we suspect happened is that when the women could not frown or make a sad expression, their brain was deprived of signals that normally reach the insula and somatosensory cortex and from there travel to language areas in the left hemisphere, where meaning is decoded.

This study helped establish that communication between the brain and body runs in both directions. There is a growing pile of evidence that supports this basic idea. For instance, several studies have had one group of participants hold a pencil horizontally with their teeth, which induces a smile, while other participants held a pencil in their lips with one end sticking out, which makes you unable to smile. (The cover story the researchers gave their volunteers was that this was a study of "psychomotoric coordination.") People were then asked to rate cartoons. Those whose pencil holding made them smile thought the cartoons were significantly funnier than did participants who were prevented from smiling. But how important is this bidirectionality?

Asthma: A Model for Mind-Brain-Body Connections

One day in 2000 I was sitting with several of my students and colleagues in our lab conference room in the psychology building, brainstorming about a "good" illness to study that would help to reveal connections between Emotional Styles and health. We had three requirements. First, it had to be an illness with known biological effects that could be measured objectively; the symptoms couldn't be simply subjective distress. Second, there had to be strong evidence that psychosocial factors, particularly stressful life events, modulate the course or symptoms of the illness; that would suggest that the brain's emotion circuits and thus Emotional Style must play a role in the illness. Third, it should be a disease that is a major public health concern and that places high demands on our health-care system; that way, anything we discovered about interventions targeting Emotional Style and/or the brain's emotion circuits would have the potential to offer significant real-world benefits. We came up with an illness that I never imagined I would study: asthma. But in science, you never know where the work will take you.

Since neither I nor anyone else in my lab knew much about asthma, we had to find someone who did. One of the joys of doing science is interacting with people way outside your own discipline, and fortunately the University of Wisconsin, Madison, is full of them—including a world-class asthma research group. Lucky for me, physician-scientist William Busse, one of the world's foremost asthma experts and the director of a huge study of asthma in inner cities, was intrigued by my proposal that we collaborate. He had previously conducted research showing that stress can exacerbate asthma symptoms, and immediately understood that the brain *must* be involved. Stressful events, after all, are complex things. Understanding and feeling stressed out by something like getting an audit letter from the IRS, or checking your 401(k) balance online and seeing that it has shrunk, or not being able to get a meeting with your boss while rumors of layoffs are circulating requires interpretation by the brain.

In his earlier asthma study, William had teamed up with psychologist Chris Coe, who studies psychoneuroimmunology, the relationship between mind, brain, and immune system. They recruited twenty undergraduates, all of whom had asthma, and exposed them to a small dose of an inhaled allergen (either ragweed, dust mites, or cat dander, whichever triggered the greatest decline in lung function during a screening test) twice during a semester: once when things were not very stressful and again just before final exams. The students also provided sputum samples, which contain molecules produced when the lungs are inflamed—as happens when an asthmatic inhales an allergen—and thus are a reliable marker of lung inflammation. Before the students' exposure to the ragweed, dust mites, or cat dander, their load of inflammatory molecules was the same during finals as it had been earlier in the semester. But after exposure to the allergen, inflammatory markers in the sputum were 27 percent higher during finals than they were during the low-stress period—even though the two allergen exposures were identical. Stress, it seems, significantly worsens the physiological response to an allergen.

The exact mechanism by which this occurs is still not completely understood, but one very recent finding suggests that it involves cortisol. Stress increases levels of cortisol, which at first glance might be beneficial to an asthmatic: Cortisol inhibits inflammation. Then how can lung inflammation increase despite higher levels of cortisol? Because immune cells become less responsive to cortisol, and the normal inflammation-inhibiting function of cortisol is disrupted. Unfortunately, few physicians who treat asthma ever consider the possibility that anything above the lung plays a role in the disease.

This and other related studies clearly indicate that although asthma is commonly thought of as an illness of the airways and, possibly, the immune system, it has a strong emotional—and therefore neurological—component as well. The stress felt by students cramming for finals triggers more severe asthma symptoms if they get exposed to an allergen. Along with other similar observations of stress exacerbating asthma symptoms, this shows that the brain is communicating with the airways and lungs. We therefore decided to explore the relationship between stress and asthma symptoms—or, more specifically, to see which patterns of brain activity affect airway obstruction and lung inflammation in asthma.

To do this, the first thing we needed was a good way to induce stress. We came up with an asthma version of the well-known Stroop task, which I mentioned previously. Originally developed in 1935, the Stroop test consists of names of colors printed either in the hue that matches them or in a different one: *Green* is in either green ink or red, for instance. The task is to name the color of the ink without saying the word. It takes longer to name the color when it is dissonant from the word than when it matches—longer to come up with "red" when the word is *green* than it does to come up with "green" for *green*. More recent versions of the Stroop have participants name the color in which emotion-laden words are written. This research has shown that among patients with anxiety disorders, for example, naming the color in which words like *anxious, nervous,* and *jittery* are written takes longer than naming the color in which nonemotional words like *house* or *curtain* are written. In both the original Stroop and the modified version, the reason it takes longer to name the color ink is that we cannot help but read the word; that interferes with naming the color.

For our first asthma study, we recruited six patients from the Madison area. When they came into the lab, we explained that they would inhale either of three substances: simple saline, which does not ordinarily induce asthma symptoms such as coughing and wheezing; methacholine, which as a smooth muscle constrictor produces the chest tightness often associated with an asthma attack but does not trigger an inflammatory response in the lungs; or an allergen (we used *eau de* dust mite or ragweed). Neither the spritzer nor the spritzee—the scientist or the participant—knew what the spritz contained, since we didn't want the mere thought of an allergen to influence a participant's reaction. A few hours after inhaling the unknown compound, each participant slid into the MRI tube.

Once he was inside, we turned on a screen built into the ceiling of the tube and, using an audio hookup to headphones we had him wear, asked him to begin the Stroop task. We chose a Stroop test with asthma-related words like *wheeze, suffocate,* and *tightness,* as well as generic negative words such as *hate, angry,* and *anxious.* As usual, the words appeared in different colors and the participants were instructed to identify the color (rather than having them call out the answer, we asked them to press different buttons for different colors; talking can mess up MRI measurements). We did this on three separate occasions, one month apart, so we could get data after the participants had inhaled each of the three substances.

Melissa Rosenkranz, a talented graduate student, took the lead. As we sat together in the control room watching the data flow in from the first participant, we could sense we were getting something. When the asthmatics saw asthma words like *wheeze,* two regions of their brain showed heightened activation: the insula, which monitors the condition of the body and also sends signals to the visceral organs during emotion; and the anterior cingulate cortex, which plays a key role in monitoring the environment and initiating action to facilitate goal-directed behavior. What's more, the extra activation in these regions was greater in response to asthma words after the participant had inhaled the allergen than when he had inhaled saline or methacholine. The asthmatics who displayed the highest levels of activation in these regions in response to asthma words also had the worst lung inflammation (which we measured twenty-four hours after the fMRI scan, when they returned to the lab). In fact, *only* those asthmatics who showed the strong brain response to the asthma words had the serious inflammation.

What these findings show is that for someone with asthma, words like *wheeze* and *suffocate* are so emotionally charged that they elicit a cascade of activity, first in the brain and then in the body. What we suspect occurs is that asthmatics differ in their sensitivity to asthma-related stressors. Those asthmatics who are most sensitive fall toward the Slow to Recover end of the Resilience style: They are walloped by setbacks and struggle to return to their previous emotional state. When they are presented with antigen, the antigen sensitizes their brain and causes them to be hyperresponsive to asthma-relevant stressors such as words like *tightness* and *suffocate*. Their response to these emotional words activates the insula and anterior cingulate cortex, which further exacerbates the inflammatory response in the lung through pathways from these brain regions to systems that release molecules that regulate inflammation, such as cortisol.

Resilience is only one of the dimensions of Emotional Style that play a role in asthma. So does Self-Awareness. As you recall from chapter 4, the brain basis for this dimension is centered on the insula. In asthmatics who are particularly susceptible to stress, the insula is overactivated, particularly by asthma-relevant stimuli such as words like *wheeze* and *suffocate*. This overactivation of the insula might provoke a decrease in lung function, which suggests that becoming *less* Self-Aware might be beneficial to someone with asthma.

These new findings on asthma suggest the possibility of using a novel approach to treatment. Since the brain is very clearly involved in modulating the inflammatory response in the lung (the key underlying process in asthma), if we can alter the neural circuitry involved, we might be able to ameliorate some of the symptoms and improve the course of the illness. In chapter 11, I will describe how we can change the brain by transforming our mind through methods such as meditation; as it happens, some of the key circuits implicated in asthma, involving the insula and anterior cingulate cortex, are the ones affected by meditation. For instance, we have trained people in mindfulness meditation, a technique in which you observe your own thoughts and feelings moment to moment and without judgment, from the perspective of a third party. Perhaps mindfulness training will allow an asthmatic to read an asthma-related word such as *wheeze* without emotional reaction. If so, it might prevent the word from triggering the physiological events that lead to an asthma attack. In this way, mental training would alter patterns of brain activity, which may produce real results relevant to health and disease.

Emotional Styles and Immunity

As you can see from these examples, there is compelling evidence that the state of your mind affects the state of your body and, more specifically, that emotions influence physiology and therefore health. But what more can we say about the specific Emotional Styles and health?

As you remember, the discovery that launched my quest to understand the brain bases for individual differences in what I would come to call Emotional Style was the asymmetry of activation in the prefrontal cortex, in which greater left than right activation is associated with positive emotions and greater right than left activation is associated with negative emotions. In the course of that research, I had become aware of some obscure studies showing that, in mice, damage to either the left or right cortical region has dramatically different effects on immune function. Damage to the left hemisphere, which in humans has been associated with depression, resulted in depressed immune function. But damage to the right cortical regions did not. Inspired by this finding, I decided to see if people might show the same basic effect. That is, might reducing activity in the left side of the brain cause not only mental illness such as depression but also somatic illness?

I therefore got back in touch with twenty undergraduates who had participated in some of my earlier studies and had been found to have dramatically lopsided frontal activity, either extreme left-sided prefrontal activation or extreme right-sided prefrontal activation. When they arrived at the lab, we took blood samples and analyzed them for natural killer (NK) cells, a type of white blood cell that constitutes a major component of our innate immune system, attacking tumors and killing cells that have been infected by viruses. What we found was that the frontal asymmetry pattern that characterizes a more positive emotional style—left frontal activation—was associated with higher NK cell activity. Participants with high left frontal activation had upwards of 50 percent higher activity than those with high right frontal activation. This finding was remarkably similar to what had been observed in the mice. Since twenty is a fairly small number of participants, I repeated this study several years later, with essentially the same results: greater left frontal activity brings greater NK cell activity.

But does greater NK activity translate into anything meaningful? I wanted to test a more clearly valid measure of immune function, and in 2003 I realized that testing how people respond to a vaccine (which indicates whether they are developing immunity) was an elegant way to do this. Melissa Rosenkranz, a graduate student in my lab, tackled the question of whether there is an association between prefrontal activity and immune response to a vaccine. She recruited fifty-two middle-aged men and women in the middle of flu season, which in Wisconsin runs from late autumn into spring. The first time the participants came to the lab, she measured their brain electrical activity to obtain their frontal asymmetry status. Then Barbara, a research nurse, gave all the participants an influenza vaccine and asked them to return three times: in two weeks, four weeks, and twenty-six weeks. At each subsequent visit we drew blood and analyzed it for influenza antibodies, an indication of whether the person had responded as intended to the flu shot.

The data for this study took a long time to collect, since we took the final blood samples six months after giving the vaccine. And analyzing the EEG data took nine months, which can be frustrating for a young scientist. So Melissa's excitement when she finally got the results was understandable. One afternoon she burst into my office, interrupting a meeting, and blurted out her findings: People with greater left-frontal activation, associated with a more positive emotional style, had the strongest immune response. The antibody levels of the most extreme left-siders averaged four times that of the most extreme right-siders. That is a huge difference and almost surely clinically significant. The greater the antibody level, the less likely you are to catch the flu.

The Heart-Brain Connection

I mentioned at the beginning of this chapter that scientists can be very insular, having little interest in exploring phenomena outside their own narrow specialty. I encountered something of this mind-set in the late 1990s, when biomedical researchers were developing ways to assess heart function through MRI rather than more invasive methods such as angiography, in which a catheter is threaded directly into the heart. When I heard about this, it occurred to me that I already had a steady parade of volunteers sliding into the MRI tube in our first-floor laboratory, for experiments in which we probed the brain activity that accompanies various emotional states. I thought, *Why not look at other organs that may also change during emotional states?*

When I approached some university colleagues who were among the leading lights in the development of MRI for probing cardiac function and described what I had in mind—using MRI in healthy people to see how psychological states such as emotions affect the heart—they were very skeptical. Cardiac MRI is designed to assess disease, they reminded me. They couldn't imagine that emotions would influence the heart sufficiently to show up on a cardiac MRI. That made me worry that our usual methods for inducing emotion in the laboratory might not be powerful enough to produce a change that the cardiac MRI could detect. So, for the first time in my research career, I decided I would have to induce fear not by presenting pictures or film clips, as I usually did, but by threatening my volunteers with an electric shock.

Psychologists have long used electric shock in both animals and humans to study fear and learning. For instance, a standard experiment is to shock a rat when it is exposed to a stimulus such as a simple tone or a colored light. The rat learns to associate the stimulus with the shock, and as a result every time the stimulus occurs, the rat's heart rate soars and it tries to escape the shock. In people, countless experiments have used electric shock, including those in which anxious patients and healthy controls were the rats, with the result that anxious patients learned to associate the stimulus with the shock faster than healthy people did. Perhaps the most famous study of electric shock only pretended to use it: the Stanley Milgram experiment in which volunteers were told they had to administer shocks to unseen partners whenever they got an answer wrong, increasing the voltage for each wrong answer. (There were no actual shocks; the idea was to see if ordinary people could be coerced by authority figures—the scientists—to torture innocent strangers. Answer: Yes.)

I was always wary of using electric shocks because they are such an unnatural stimulus, not to mention that it didn't seem ethical to shock research participants when we had other ways of inducing fear or anxiety. However, given my colleagues' skepticism about whether the usual ways of inducing negative emotions would produce a measurable effect on the heart, I decided to go for it.

For the experiment, I used what's called in the trade the "threat of shock" procedure more than actual shocks. We recruited twenty-three college students through advertisements around campus and explained that they would be put into the MRI tube and see, projected on the ceiling, simple geometric shapes such as a diamond and a circle. One shape—the diamond— meant that they might receive an electric shock, while the other meant all would be well. Just so they knew what they were in for, we administered a mild shock for twenty milliseconds (that's one-fiftieth of a second), which felt like the zap you experience if you've ever touched a fully charged nine-volt battery to your tongue. Then they slid into the MRI tube and began watching the ceiling.

Standing in the control room as real-time measurements of brain activity poured in, I was struck by the large differences in the pattern of neural activation when people saw the "shock alert!" diamond compared with the "don't worry" circle. I was zeroing in on several parts of the brain that I knew should be activated by fear, such as the amygdala, insula, and prefrontal cortex. But it isn't surprising that feeling threatened has a different neural profile than feeling safe. As the heart readings also came in—we were measuring contractility, or the strength with which the heart beats, in particular—I could see immediately that, at least for some participants, emotions had reached down into the chest and wreaked havoc. Contractility is influenced by the sympathetic nervous system, which is the key constituent of the fight-or-flight response and has been implicated in stress and distress. The stronger the brain activation in three key regions—a sector of the right prefrontal cortex, the insula, and the amygdala—the stronger the cardiac contractility. In response to the diamond threat cue, some people had little change in their contractility while others had a dramatic change.

We were able to sort out who was who by looking at their brains. More than 40 percent of the person-to-person variation in cardiac contractility was accounted for by how strongly the insula and the prefrontal cortex responded to the shape that was the harbinger of threat. This heightened brain activity was racing down the highways of the sympathetic nervous system and making the heart pump harder. Such differences in emotional style are likely to be consequential for health when they are played out over a long period of time.

The Embodied Mind

The mind is "embodied" in the sense that it exists within the body—specifically, in the three pounds of tofulike tissue we call the brain—and engages in bidirectional communication with it, so that the state of the mind influences the body, and the state of the body influences the mind. Emotions, too, are embodied, and given their power to affect physiology outside the skull they are arguably the most embodied form of mental activity. The brain circuits that underlie Emotional Styles have extensive two-way connections with the immune system, the endocrine system, and the autonomic nervous system. Through traffic in one direction, from brain to body, the mind influences our health. This suggests that knowing someone's Emotional Style may be as important to a health-care provider, in terms of assessing health risks, as knowing whether the patient smokes, and that altering your Emotional Style can be beneficial to physiological systems and thus overall health. Through traffic in the other direction, from body to brain, changes in our patterns of movement can affect how our mind processes emotional information. That has implications beyond warning Botox users that paralyzing some of their facial muscles runs the risk of limiting their emotional range. It also suggests that the body can become an ally in transforming emotion, meaning practices that emphasize the body, such as hatha yoga, have the potential to modulate emotion. This research is barely off the ground, but there are tantalizing hints about how this body-to-brain connection might work.

CHAPTER 7

■ ■ ■

Normal and Abnormal, and When "Different" Becomes Pathological

What is emotionally normal, anyway? When I introduced the six dimensions of Emotional Style in the introduction, I hope I made clear that there is no single ideal style. In fact, I will go further and say that not only is no particular spot on the spectrum of Emotional Styles superior to any other, but that civilization could never have advanced to where we are today without people who fall at many different points along each dimension.

If you like that iPads, cell phones, online banking, Second Life, Facebook, and Halo exist, then you should be glad that there are people who prefer to interact more with machines than with other individuals—people who likely fall toward the Puzzled end of the Social Intuition spectrum. If you're relieved that political assassinations don't happen more often than they do, then you should be glad that Secret Service agents fall toward the Socially Intuitive end of the Social Intuition style, making them extremely sensitive to subtle, nonverbal cues in the environment. If you like that modern society has successful teachers and effective leaders, then you should be glad that there are people who fall toward the Fast to Recover end of the Resilience style, the Positive end of the Outlook style, the Socially Intuitive end of the Social Intuition style (teachers and leaders need to be sensitive to the cues of those around them), and the Tuned In end of the Social Context style (they need to be sensitive to the niceties of the social environment to respond appropriately in a given situation). In short, variations in Emotional Style serve our society well by equipping different people with different, complementary strengths.

Sometimes, however, a style can be sufficiently extreme that it interferes with daily functioning. When it does, it crosses over into pathology. This is no different from measures of physical function. Blood pressure, cholesterol levels, heart rate, and other physiological measures range along a continuum just as the dimensions of the Emotional Styles do. For all of these, there is a cutpoint beyond which a value is considered pathological because it is associated with illness, such as a greater risk of stroke or cardiovascular disease. The boundary between health and disease is somewhat arbitrary and can change as biomedical research advances (witness the decrease in the cholesterol level considered healthy). In general, however, that boundary is where the physiological measure results in an impairment to daily living. It may be interesting to have an academic argument about what's a healthy lung capacity, but I think we'd all agree that when you can't climb stairs without feeling too winded to continue, you've crossed the boundary into the pathological.

The same is true for Emotional Style. When your Resilience style is so Slow to Recover that the slightest setback tips you into another acute episode of panic or anxiety, it has become pathological. When your Outlook style is so Negative that the absence of joy in your life makes you seriously consider ending it all, it has become pathological. When your Social Intuition style is so Puzzled that you have difficulty understanding basic social interactions and cannot form close relationships, it has become pathological—and may even fall along the autism spectrum. When your Self-Awareness style is so Self-Opaque that you are unable to perceive when your stress level begins skyrocketing, you have no clue that you need to take steps to reduce stress, which (as I described in chapter 6) increases your risk of illness. When your Sensitivity to Context style is so Tuned Out from your surroundings that you mistake the siren of an ambulance for a medevac unit on the battlefield, it has become pathological, maybe even sliding into post-traumatic stress disorder. When your Attention style is so Unfocused that you can't complete even simple tasks or learn what you need in order to succeed academically or professionally, it has become pathological and could even indicate full-blown attention deficit/hyperactivity disorder.

For some of these dimensions, the opposite end can be pathological, too.

For example, if your Outlook style sustains the Positive too much, you might be at risk for bipolar disorder or variants of mania marked by inappropriate positive emotion. You can be so excessively Self-Aware and flooded by sensations from your body that you become prone to panic attacks. And you can be so Focused that you miss something, or someone, that requires your attention.

As you might have guessed from these examples, virtually all the major forms of psychiatric disorder involve some dysregulation of emotion. You can therefore think of Emotional Style as shaping how vulnerable someone will be to mental illness. Although Emotional Style cannot, in itself, *cause* mental illness, it does interact with other factors to determine whether or not a person might develop one. Disturbances in emotional function lie at the core of mood and anxiety disorders, for instance, which is not surprising: In mood disorders such as depression, people are unable to maintain positive feelings such as happiness or even interest, while in generalized anxiety disorder and social anxiety disorder they have a hard time turning off negative emotion once it is turned on. But, perhaps more surprisingly, emotional disturbances are also central to schizophrenia and autism. Schizophrenia is often marked by anhedonia, the inability to derive pleasure from normal activities. And people with autism have such difficulty interpreting innocuous social cues, such as the expression on a stranger's face, that they take them as a threat, retreating further and further into their own world until even the entreaties of those closest to them cannot coax them out.

Neurally Based Psychiatry

By understanding which dimensions of Emotional Style might be implicated in particular disorders and how they might contribute to the core symptoms of the disorder, we can better appreciate the continuum between normal and abnormal. Identifying the contribution of the different dimensions to particular disorders will also help to pinpoint the underlying brain systems that contribute to each disorder and suggest new strategies to treat it by altering the Emotional Style that lies at its core. This, I am convinced, is the future of psychiatric research. Currently, clinicians assess a patient's symptoms, and if enough of them match those that characterize, say, social phobia or obsessive-compulsive disorder or bipolar disorder, then bingo—she is classified as having that disorder. The problem with this yes-or-no approach is that it fails to recognize that people vary and that the tipping point for "you have this" is arbitrary. Most important, dividing the pie into 365 distinct disorders, the number of diseases in the *Diagnostic and Statistical Manual of Mental Disorders*, or *DSM* (whose fifth edition the American Psychiatric Association plans to release in 2013, after six years of work by thousands of psychiatrists and psychologists), does not conform to how the brain functions. A better approach, and one that I have been advocating since I was president of the Society for Research in Psychopathology in 1996, is to place people along neuroscientifically grounded continua.

Let me use an example to explain how this would work. A number of psychiatric disorders involve abnormalities in the capacity to experience pleasure. Depression is the most obvious such disease, but the inability to feel joy, happiness, or contentment—anhedonia—also characterizes schizophrenia, as noted already. Many people think of this disease as being primarily marked by hallucinations and delusions, and these are indeed the so-called positive symptoms of schizophrenia, in which "positive" means that a symptom is present. But schizophrenia is also a disease of "negative" symptoms, meaning the absence of qualities that are normally present. The most striking negative symptom of schizophrenia is anhedonia. In the framework of Emotional Styles, anhedonia puts someone at the extreme Negative end of the Outlook spectrum. The Outlook style is therefore likely to play a role in schizophrenia—as well as in depression, anxiety disorders, addictive disorders, and others in which problems with positive emotions are prominent.

This chapter will consider the boundary between normal and abnormal as it applies to three dimensions of Emotional Style: Social Intuition, which plays a key role in autism; Outlook, which affects risk of depression; and Attention, which accounts for ADHD.

The Autism Spectrum

I have my daughter to thank for my interest in autism. From the moment Amelie was old enough to notice other people, which for her was not long after she was born, she was a social butterfly. That trait stood out starkly when, in high school, she tutored an eleven-year-old autistic girl named Molly for her bat mitzvah. Besides helping Molly with her Hebrew, Amelie was an important social connection for her. I will never forget attending Molly's bat mitzvah, and knowing that Amelie had played a huge role in her ability to stand in front of the entire congregation, reciting her prayers and Torah readings without flinching.

The classical description of autism includes a triad of symptoms. The first involves disturbances in social interaction, such that people with autism avoid eye contact, often do not respond to their own names, and usually appear unaware of others' feelings. The second group of symptoms centers on communication problems, such that some autistics barely speak, speak with an abnormal tone or rhythm, repeat words or phrases without knowing what they mean, or find it impossible to initiate a conversation. The third group of symptoms involves stereotyped behaviors such as performing repetitive movements (for example, hand flapping or rocking) or engaging in specific routines or rituals, such as needing to always have a sip of milk at the start of a meal and finishing the main course before touching any side dishes.

Modern research has broadened the category of autism to include the "autism spectrum," which means that there is a wide range of severity for each element of the symptom triad. Some children identified as falling on the autism spectrum merely have poor eye contact and a somewhat abnormal, flat tone to their speech, for instance. Others explode in terrified, and terrifying, paroxysms of rage if someone touches them, speaks to them, or tries to get them to make eye contact. For still others, the most visible symptom is being fixated on a specific part of a plaything, such as the wheels of a toy truck. As a result, individuals on the autism spectrum range from those who function well in society, such as the renowned animal behaviorist Temple Grandin, to those who are so functionally impaired that they cannot speak, are unable to attend school, and need constant care. Regardless of where someone falls on the autism spectrum, however, there is some impairment in social interaction and social communication.

During Amelie and Molly's tutoring sessions in our dining room, I noticed one very striking thing about Molly: her lack of eye contact. I could tell that she was paying attention to what Amelie told her, because when Amelie asked her to read lines from the Torah aloud, she clearly tried to do so. But Molly never looked at Amelie. This made me wonder whether the lack of eye contact might provide a window into the basis of autism, and how it might be related to the well-known impairments in social communication that autistic people have, such as being less able to detect irony, sarcasm, or humor. Over time, as I met other children with autism, I observed that no matter how mild or severe the disease, gaze aversion was a consistent symptom.

By this point in my research (Amelie's sessions with Molly took place in 1999), I was already formulating my theory of Emotional Style and had provisionally included Social Intuition as one of the six dimensions. It occurred to me that one of the consequences of gaze aversion would be poor social intuition. The reason is that so many of the social signals we transmit—those of interest or boredom, surprise or pleasure or trust—come from around the eyes, as the great French anatomist Duchenne, whom I introduced you to in chapter 2, argued. Because the muscles around the eyes convey true emotion, this region of the face is crucial to social communication. I knew this from some of my earliest research on emotion, when the volunteers watching amusing video clips back in my lab at SUNY Purchase had characteristic eye-muscle movements (wrinkling the corners of the eyes) that went along with their brain-activity patterns. These were the studies in which we found that true happiness, as determined by eye-crinkling smiles, is accompanied by spikes of activity in the left prefrontal region, but faked happiness, without the crinkles, is not. This study showed that only when you observe the eyes can you accurately discern that someone is experiencing a positive emotion.

This memory came rushing back to me when I saw that Molly couldn't look into Amelie's eyes. Given the prevalence of gaze aversion among children and adults who fall on the autism spectrum, I realized that they must be missing important cues about people's emotional states. They wouldn't be able to tell that a jesting, tongue-in-cheek remark like, "Gee, only a 98? I guess you didn't study very hard for that test," or "A one-carat emerald ring? I guess our anniversary doesn't mean very much to you," actually means the opposite of its literal meaning: You studied your backside off for that test and did great; this is the most wonderful gift anyone has ever given me. No wonder people with autism have such difficulty with social interaction—they can't pick up on what other people are feeling and what their words and behavior mean. This social and emotional blindness, I suspected, might not be the result of any specific deficit in emotion processing in the brain, as was widely believed. Instead, it might be the consequence of not looking at people's eyes. If non-autistic people spent a day averting their eyes from the faces of their colleagues and companions, they would miss all manner of social and emotional cues, too, and be equally perplexed by the social world around them. This suggests that if autistic people could somehow learn to look at people's eyes, without discomfort or anxiety, much of their social and emotional deficit might melt away.

That was far from the expert consensus, however. Several studies had concluded that children with autism may have a fundamental abnormality in the fusiform gyrus, the cluster of neurons located in the visual cortex in the back of the brain that perceives faces. The 1997 discovery that a region of the brain is specialized for perceiving faces—not trees, not rocks, not furniture, not food, and not any other part of the anatomy—made some sense, since faces are so important in the social lives of humans and other primates (chimps have a fusiform gyrus, too, a 2009 study found). Follow-up studies, however, found that the fusiform gyrus is not necessarily specialized for faces, but kicks into gear whenever people perceive an object that belongs to a category in which they have expertise. In auto aficionados and expert bird-watchers, for instance, the fusiform gyrus becomes active at the sight of cars and birds, respectively. That is, when a bird-watcher is shown pictures of, say, cardinals and titmice and ducks and albatross, and is asked to classify them, the fusiform gyrus lights up with activity. That's why scientists were initially misled into thinking the fusiform gyrus is specialized for face perception and only face perception: People are experts at perceiving faces and habitually try to classify them (stranger? friend?). The fusiform gyrus, studies claimed, is deficient in people with autism. When children with autism lie in an MRI tube so their brain activity can be monitored, and are presented with face discrimination tasks such as classifying whether a face depicts happiness or anger, their fusiform gyrus is much less active than it is in kids who are developing normally.

I was skeptical about pinning autism on an inherent deficit in the fusiform gyrus. Think about it: Here are kids with autism, who have terrible problems relating to other people, and a bunch of strangers are sliding them into a deafening, claustrophobia-inducing MRI tube and instructing them to perform tasks involving the perception of faces. I thought it more than likely that the kids either stared unfocused into space, trying to calm themselves, or just shut their eyes until the whole ordeal was over. If so, then of course their fusiform gyrus was quiet. Unbeknownst to the scientists (who didn't have any detectors in the MRI tube to monitor where the children were actually fixing their eyes), the autistic children may not have even been looking at the faces projected on the MRI ceiling, let alone trying to discriminate among the faces' emotions. The lack of activity in the fusiform gyrus, I suspected, did not reflect a fusiform defect; it was the result of the fact that the children were averting their eyes from the faces the scientists flashed at them. To conclude the former was analogous to saying that lack of activity in the auditory cortex is the reason your teenager cannot hear you call him for dinner, when in fact it's because he's wearing noise-canceling headphones. A lack of activity does not necessarily imply defective function; it might simply reflect a lack of input.

If You Don't Look, You Can't See

To see if my suspicion was right, my colleagues and I launched the first study examining the neural correlates of face perception in children with autism while simultaneously measuring the kids' gaze patterns. We used fiber-optic goggles to present the images we wanted the children to see; the goggles had a built-in infrared laser eye-tracking system that allowed us to monitor the children's eye movements. The task we presented was very simple, since we wanted kids at all levels of functioning to be able to do it: We projected a single face into the fiber-optic goggles for three seconds and instructed the children to press one of two buttons to indicate whether the face was emotional or neutral. Based on Duchenne's work, we knew that the children would have to look in the eye region of the face in order to make that determination.

It was a humbling experience to be sitting in the fMRI control room, monitoring the data as we collected it. As earlier studies had found, the children with autism did much more poorly on the task than did a control group of nonautistic children. The autistic children classified 85 percent of the faces correctly, compared with ninety-eight percent of the normal children. (Eighty-five percent might seem high, but keep in mind that the children in the study were functioning well enough to be able to come to our lab, interact sufficiently with strangers to follow instructions, and tolerate the tight quarters and loud banging of the MRI tube.) The autistic children also showed diminished activation in the fusiform gyrus, as other studies had found.

But there was something even more striking. As each face—some neutral, some displaying an emotion—came up through the goggles, I saw the path of the children's eyes: Many of them would look anywhere *but* the eyes of the face. When we examined the record of the autistic children's eye movements more systematically, after we had data on all thirty of them, we found that these children spent an average of 20 percent less time looking into the eyes of the faces in the pictures compared with the normally developing children. Once we took that into account, it explained almost all the variation in how activated their fusiform region was. There was nothing wrong with the autistic children's fusiform region. It was quiescent not because it was impaired but because it wasn't receiving any signals. It wasn't receiving signals because the kids averted their gaze from other people's faces and, especially, from their eyes.

This was a significant finding, disproving the conventional wisdom that autistic people are inherently neurologically impaired when it comes to perceiving faces. But another, even more important finding emerged. The brain activity of the autistic children differed from that of typically developing children in another region during the face perception task: There was greater activity in the amygdala. The amygdala, you recall, is critical for emotional learning and is a key structure in circuits important for fear and anxiety; it is responsible for perceiving threats in the environment. Many of the autistic children who could hardly look into the eyes of a face in a photo (let alone a real, live face) had sky-high levels of activity in the amygdala. The fact that amygdala activity is elevated when autistic children look at faces—even for a few fractions of a second, as in this experiment—suggests that doing so makes them profoundly uncomfortable, even fearful, and that when they look into someone's eyes their brains and bodies are flooded with messages that they interpret as threatening. Only by looking away can they stop this onslaught. Indeed, when the kids averted their gaze from the eye region of the faces (as revealed by the eye-tracking system), activation in the amygdala fell, suggesting that gaze aversion is a calming, emotion-regulating strategy to relieve anxiety and fear. By avoiding other people's eyes, the autistic child can decrease the social stimulation he finds so threatening.

If high levels of amygdala activation are uncomfortable and interpreted by the brain as signaling the presence of something threatening, as these findings suggest, then innocuous expressions on the faces of strangers and even family members are likely being interpreted as threatening. I suspect that children with autism hit upon the strategy of averting their gaze early in life. They feel anxious when they look at faces, and discover that they can relieve or avoid that anxiety by looking anywhere else.

But that relief comes at a steep cost. As a consequence of averting their gaze from the faces of other people, they miss the important social information that faces, and especially eyes, convey. Mike, an autistic fifteen-year-old who participated in our studies, confirmed this to me. He was intensely curious about our research and eager to learn more about the findings. After his session in the scanner, I asked Mike if he would be willing to come into a graduate seminar I was teaching and talk about his autism, describing what it feels like to look at other people's faces and interact socially. He happily agreed. Sitting at the table with a dozen students, I asked Mike about making eye contact. He described in poignant terms the difficulty and ridicule he encounters as a result of not looking people straight in the face. Kids at school assume he doesn't care about them because he does not look at their eyes when speaking with them. But Mike feels he has little choice. He feels abject terror, he told us, whenever he looks at faces and, especially, at eyes.

All in the Family

Autism has the strongest heritability of any neuropsychiatric disorder. The background prevalence is almost 1 percent, with current estimates of about one in 110 eight-year-old children having a diagnosis of autism spectrum disorder. But if one child in a family has autism, the likelihood that a sibling will, too, is about 3 percent—triple the background rate. Among identical twins, who have identical DNA sequences, if one twin has autism, then the other does in 63 to 98 percent of the cases (the range reflects what different studies have found). Clearly, then, autism has a genetic component. No "autism genes" have been definitively identified, although there are a number of suspects, and it seems clear that many genes must be present to cause the disease. This suggests that when someone inherits fewer than the threshold number of autism genes needed to develop the full-blown disease, he might still show some symptoms of it.

To see if this is so, we conducted a study of the siblings of children with autism—brothers and sisters who did not fall even at the mild end of the autism spectrum. Yet they, too, had unusual eye-tracking patterns. They did not avert their gazes from other people's faces and eyes as assiduously as their autistic siblings did. But upon close examination, they exhibited a pattern of eye tracking and brain activation that was in between that of their affected siblings and typically developing children. That is, activity in their amygdala jumped when they looked at faces. It didn't jump as high as their autistic siblings' did, but it jumped nonetheless. When they looked at faces, their gaze fell on the eye region much less often than did the gaze of typically developing children. This finding reinforces the idea that underlies the theory of Emotional Style: Social Intuition varies along a continuum, and the dividing line between normal and abnormal is somewhat arbitrary.

Just how arbitrary became clear as we scrutinized these data. Most of us think we know the difference between health and sickness, between normal and pathological. I did, too, believing that although behavioral symptoms might fool us, brain-activity patterns—which have been specifically linked to more and more psychiatric illnesses, promising to serve as signatures of those illnesses—can be trusted. As I looked more closely at the data on autistic and typically developing children who were shown images of faces, I saw that the amount of amygdala activity in the autistic children was indeed greater, on average, than it was in healthy children who looked at faces. But the activity in the autistic kids varied enormously. And the amount of amygdala activity in some typically developing children was as great as in the autistic children.

It was at this point that I realized that the dividing line between normal and abnormal is problematic. Many of the language and social symptoms of autism—and the brain processes that underlie these symptoms—are present throughout the population. People who do not have autism but cannot stand to look in people's eyes are sometimes labeled "social phobic." But this label, I argue, does not describe a discrete, easily identified illness. It is just the far end of a range. This shows that there is no magic cut-point on any of the dimensions of Emotional Style that marks the division between normalcy and pathology.

A Brain Taxonomy of Depression

Most people think of depression as the pervasive, unshakable presence of sadness and even despair. That certainly describes many of those who suffer from this cruel disease. But more recent research has identified other hallmarks of depression, most notably the inability to experience pleasure and other positive emotions, such as satisfaction, joy, and pride. One consequence of the inability to feel these positive emotions is, not surprisingly, difficulties in planning, anticipating the future, and performing goal-directed action. If you can't imagine that a particular action will bring you happiness or even a sense of accomplishment, you understandably don't have much incentive to plan it, let alone do it.

All these symptoms of depression reflect aberrant patterns of activity in the prefrontal cortex and other brain regions. One of my earliest findings, as I described in chapter 2, was that people suffering from depression show much higher right-side than left-side activation of the prefrontal cortex, whereas healthy people show higher left than right activation. (And as I'll discuss in chapter 10, some of the Olympic athletes of well-being—Buddhist monks—have off-the-chart left-side activation.) But more recently, in studies of scores of patients with depression, it has become clear to me that "depression" is not one single thing like, say, rheumatoid arthritis. In other words, there are many ways to be depressed. It turns out that there are almost as many species of depression as there are of beetles, each form of which (depression, not beetles) has a characteristic pattern of brain activity. This suggests that different subgroups might benefit from different treatments.

- One distinct group of depressed patients is those who have difficulty recovering from adversity. Once something bad happens, they are thrown off course for a long time. They fall at the Slow to Recover end of the Resilience style, reflecting lower levels of left-side prefrontal activation. They have difficulty turning off negative emotions once they are turned on.

• Another subgroup of people with depression—again, not all—is those who fall toward the Tuned Out end of the Sensitivity to Context dimension. They have difficulty regulating their emotions in a context-appropriate way. For example, if they are wary and bashful in novel situations or around unfamiliar people, which is pretty normal, they may overgeneralize to familiar situations, and their wariness and shyness would persist. People with this Emotional Style act as formally and reticently with friends as they do with family. This prevents them from having rewarding social interactions, which tips them into depression. Another manifestation of being Tuned Out to social context: A supervisor at work treats you as if you cannot do anything right. Half the time she chastises you for engaging in too much small talk with customers; the other half of the time, when you have dialed back your chattiness, she berates you for being too terse. Not surprisingly, you are perpetually on edge, sure that you will make a false step no matter what you do. If you have difficulty aligning your emotions with social context, even when you are at home or among friends, you find yourself shot through with anxiety, worried about saying something wrong. Again, this puts you at risk for depression. In this subgroup, MRIs have found that the hippocampus is smaller than it is in healthy people. That makes sense: The hippocampus is a key brain region for processing context.

• A third subgroup of people with depression is those who are completely unable to sustain any positive emotion, be it excitement or happiness or hope. In contrast to emotionally healthy people who get some good news in the morning—a friend is giving him tickets to the sold-out concert!—and likely feel "up" for several hours afterward, these depressed patients show no such afterglow. They fall at the Negative pole of the Outlook dimension; their inability to maintain any positive emotion means they can never savor life's ups. Many of these patients also fall at the Slow to Recover end of the Resilience dimension. (Not all do so; the two dimensions are independent. Many people who are unable to sustain positive emotion are Fast to Recover from adversity, while some who are great at maintaining an emotional high after a positive experience nevertheless are Slow to Recover when they experience a setback.) The double hit of an inability to sustain positive emotions and an inability to shake off setbacks is a recipe for depression.

Depression and the Outlook Dimension

This last group, those who have difficulty sustaining positive emotions, has been the focus of my research on depression. Curiously, although depression is generally viewed as an emotional or mood disorder, very little research has actually investigated emotional processing in patients with depression. That reflects, I think, a "not my job" attitude in both psychiatry and psychology. The former does not study normal emotion; in particular, it does not study positive emotions. The latter does, but psychologists who study normal emotion seldom interact with those who study psychopathology. As a result, there has been very little research on abnormalities in the processes that generate and sustain positive emotions. That's where I plunged in.

In one of my earliest studies, described in chapter 4, we showed depressed patients and healthy controls one- to two-minute clips from comedy movies chosen to induce a feeling of happiness. Much to my surprise, immediately after watching the clips the depressed patients reported about the same average level of positive emotion—happiness, contentment, enthusiasm—on a five-point scale as the controls. Depressed people had just as much capacity for positive emotions as the healthy controls did.

Years later, I went back to the raw data from this study, still bothered by what I regarded as this anomalous finding. By then, my work on Emotional Styles had turned up the fact that people vary in how long they are able to sustain positive emotions. This became the basis for the Outlook style, with its extremes of Positive types, who are able to keep the flame of happiness burning like a Boy Scout nursing the embers of a fire, and Negative types, in whom the fire of joy is quickly doused by a sudden downpour. I therefore examined these old data more carefully, paying particular attention to the video records of the participants' facial expressions, which provide a real-time readout of their emotional state. This time, I saw that although depressed patients showed flashes of happiness in response to the comedy clips, they couldn't sustain it. The expression of positive emotions on their faces vanished quickly, rather than lingering as it did in healthy controls.

Debra, a depressed patient in one of our studies, captured the essence of this trait when she described her feelings at a dinner party at the home of a good friend. When she first arrived and greeted the hostess, Debra told me, she felt a genuine burst of happiness. But once everyone sat down to eat, her feelings began to shift: Her initial happiness vanished, and she felt the black abyss of depression yawning before her. By the time the main course arrived, the food had completely lost any taste for her, and she could hardly take a bite. She got not even the tiniest frisson of pleasure from either the other guests or the food, and she wanted to bolt from the party as soon as possible.

What might have been happening in Debra's brain during this tectonic shift in mood? In a recent experiment, mentioned in chapter 4, we trained depressed patients and healthy controls to perform what's called cognitive reappraisal. The technique involves thinking about a stimulus (we showed the participants images chosen to induce a sense of happiness) in such a way as to enhance the emotional response it elicits. In the case of happiness producing pictures, for instance, we instructed the participants to imagine that the joyous events they depicted were happening to themselves or to loved ones. When they saw a picture of a smiling mother embracing her grinning child, the participants were encouraged to imagine themselves or their loved ones in the picture. Once they understood cognitive reappraisal, we put the participants in the MRI tube and projected seventy-two such pictures, one at a time, and instructed them to cognitively enhance their emotional responses.

For about the first half of the pictures, the brains of the depressed patients and healthy controls responded almost identically when they tried to cognitively enhance their response to the pictures. In both, activation increased in the nucleus accumbens, a brain region associated with positive emotion and motivation. This area is studded with receptors for the neurotransmitter dopamine, which has been implicated in motivating a person to seek goals and rewards; and for endogenous opiates, the molecules of pleasure and other positive emotions. During the second half of the slide show, however, the pattern was very different. The healthy, control participants continued to show high levels of activation in the nucleus accumbens. Their response actually increased over time, as if the experience of turbocharging their feeling of happiness reinforced itself in a positive-feedback loop. But in the depressed patients, activity in the nucleus accumbens declined substantially during the second half of the picture show. They were unable to sustain their positive emotions—just as Debra had been unable to sustain hers. *That* is what happened in Debra's brain when her initial feelings of happiness and engagement at the dinner vanished like a well-received soup course: Activity in her nucleus accumbens fell off a cliff.

Like Debra, the participants in our study felt the consequences of that drop-off in activity. We asked them to rate how well adjectives such as *happy, energetic, excited, proud,* and *interested* described them—from not at all to extremely well. The more sustained the activation in the nucleus accumbens, the more positive emotion people reported. This, then, is the brain basis for the form of depression characterized by an inability to sustain positive emotion: The nucleus accumbens fails to sustain its activity, probably because of a malfunction in the connections between it and the prefrontal cortex. As a result, the nucleus accumbens initially snaps into action but peters out very quickly, and positive emotions fade away. This is the signature of the extreme Negative pole of the Outlook dimension as described in chapter 4.

No brain region is an island: There is massive connectivity among various regions, though of course a given region has more connections to some than to others. With fMRI, we can not only identify which regions show increased activity during tasks but also see how strongly different areas are connected to other areas functionally, by determining the correlation between the fMRI signals in two or more regions. (Basically, if two areas "light up" in concert more than most other pairs of regions do, there is a good chance that they are functionally connected, with activity in one causing activity in the other.) We therefore used the fMRI scans to map the functional connections that were specifically engaged during cognitive enhancement of pleasure.

What we saw was that a region in the prefrontal cortex called the middle prefrontal gyrus, which is involved in planning and goal-directed behavior, was strongly connected to the nucleus accumbens during this task. That is, when the middle prefrontal gyrus became active, the nucleus accumbens did too. And just as activity in the nucleus accumbens alone fell off in depressed patients, the connectivity between it and the middle prefrontal gyrus also diminished as the experiment went on. At first, both the healthy controls and the depressed patients showed strong connectivity between these regions. The controls maintained that connectivity, but in the depressed patients it began to wane. What we think happened is that although the middle prefrontal gyrus remained active, it stopped sending signals to the nucleus accumbens. It was like one half of a sleepy couple, who keeps elbowing the other to keep him awake and eventually tires of it—but remains awake herself.

This was an exciting finding because it suggested that the reason activation in the nucleus accumbens declined in the depressed patients was that the connection from the prefrontal cortex, which directs activity in other parts of the brain, was malfunctioning. The patients consciously tried to enhance their positive emotion but couldn't. Just as you might try your best to hit a golf ball straight down the fairway, if the critical connections between motor cortex and muscles are not there to enable a good swing, it's not going to happen. Without strong connections between the prefrontal cortex and the nucleus accumbens, you cannot sustain positive emotions and are at risk for tipping into depression.

The Way Forward

The reason I have been so determined to identify the brain activation patterns that underlie different mental disorders has nothing to do with adding to the long list of neural correlates that have become so popular with the advent of neuroimaging—that is, the patterns of brain activity that arise when people experience a particular feeling, think a particular thought, or engage in any other activity that involves the mind. All of that is fascinating and important, but it is only the first step. The ultimate goal is what I call neurally inspired behavioral therapy. The "neurally inspired" part means that the therapy would alter the aberrant brain activity associated with the mental illness. The "behavioral" part refers to the hope that this can be achieved not through medication but through mental training, cognitive-behavior therapy, and other interventions that essentially teach people to think about their thoughts in a different and hopefully beneficial way.

Neurally inspired therapy of all kinds, not just neurally inspired *behavioral* therapy, is still in its infancy but has scored enough preliminary success to make me believe we may be on to something. Let me give you some examples, from my work as well as that of other scientists.

To be sure that faulty connections between the frontal cortex and nucleus accumbens were causing the inability to sustain positive emotions, rather than just being innocent bystanders, I studied what happens when people with depression undergo successful therapy. We recruited twenty people with depression and, after measuring their brain function with fMRI, treated them with standard antidepressant medication for eight weeks. Some patients reported significantly more positive emotion at the end of the eight weeks, while others showed little improvement—a pattern that is typical of response to antidepressants, which help some patients but not others. But what we cared about was this: When the patients who reported more positive emotions tried to cognitively enhance the contentment they felt while looking at happy pictures, they had a substantial increase in sustained activation of the nucleus accumbens and in that region's connectivity with the prefrontal cortex. In other words, the pattern of brain activity—a quiescent nucleus accumbens and little connectivity between the nucleus accumbens and the prefrontal cortex—that characterizes an inability to sustain positive emotion reverted to the healthier pattern in people who responded to antidepressant treatment. This suggests that when the drugs work, they do so by targeting the circuitry that sustains positive emotion, perhaps by supporting signaling between the prefrontal cortex and the nucleus accumbens. Why they have this beneficial effect on some patients but not on others remains a mystery, however. We are now in the process of determining whether standard nonpharmacological therapies—cognitive therapy and interpersonal therapy—have similar effects, at least for certain depressed patients.

One of the most promising forms of neurally based therapy arises from my basic discovery about the patterns of brain activity that underlie depression:

- People with higher left than right prefrontal activity feel a greater sense of well-being and contentment, while those who have higher right than left prefrontal activity often suffer from depression. In addition, people who have greater baseline levels of left prefrontal activation score high on something called behavioral activation, which is a measure of the strength of what psychologists have called approach motivation. People with high behavioral activation scores strongly agree with statements such as "When I get something I want, I feel excited and energized" and "When I want something, I usually go all out to get it."

• People who have greater baseline levels of right prefrontal activation score high on behavioral inhibition, which is a measure of anxiety and the propensity to "shut down" in the face of adversity. Behaviorally inhibited people agree strongly with such statements as "I worry about making mistakes" and "Criticism or scolding hurts me quite a bit."

The concepts of behavioral activation and behavioral inhibition were originally introduced by British neuroscientist Jeffrey Gray and refer to systems in the brain that are associated with approach and withdrawal behavior, respectively. Behavioral activation therapy teaches patients to approach new situations, even if they are vaguely threatening, rather than avoiding difficult situations. It also teaches patients to identify activities that bring them satisfaction and are consistent with long-term goals. For instance, a patient rates the degree of pleasure and accomplishment she feels during specific activities, perhaps saying that she very much enjoys reading, socializing with a small group of close friends, and doing volunteer work at a thrift shop. The therapist would then help and encourage the patient to establish and maintain regular routines that encompass these activities rather than leave them to chance, so instead of the patient calling friends or going down to the thrift shop only when she feels the desire to do so, she makes a strict schedule, programming it into her phone calendar or otherwise holding herself to "Thursday lunch with friends" and "volunteer Tuesday morning," for instance. Finally, the therapist helps the patient let go of ruminative thoughts such as "I am a bad person" or "I fail at everything I try" by challenging her with counterexamples from her life: "You graduated from college!" "You got a job despite the lousy economy!" "The intern at work was practically in tears, so grateful was he for your mentoring!" Whatever works.

Behavioral activation therapy has shown real promise. In a large randomized control trial, 188 patients with major depressive disorder received antidepressant medication, cognitive therapy, or behavioral activation therapy. Of these, 106 patients were successfully treated, their depression lifting after sixteen weeks of treatment. Initial response rates are only the tip of the iceberg when it comes to evaluating treatments for depression, however. Even more important is whether the improvement lasts. The scientists therefore followed the patients for a full year. The patients treated with medication had the most relapses, with 59 percent suffering another acute episode of depression after they stopped taking the drugs. Patients who had received cognitive therapy or behavioral activation therapy had a rate of relapse between 40 and 50 percent. These findings indicate that not only are these psychological treatments effective, but they are more effective at minimizing relapse than medication—and they are less costly.

And now we have hints that behavioral activation therapy might be the kind of neurally inspired treatment I described earlier. In a 2009 study, scientists performed fMRIs before and after treatment with behavioral activation therapy. They examined neural responses to a rewarding gambling task during conditions in which participants were expecting to receive a reward. After twelve weeks of treatment, 75 percent of patients showed a marked reduction in depressive symptoms. They also showed an increase in activation in the striatum, a brain region that includes the nucleus accumbens. The findings suggest that training designed to increase engagement with rewarding stimuli and decrease avoidance behaviors leads to marked changes in brain circuits important for sustained experience of positive emotion. These new findings hold out the promise that behavioral activation therapy may specifically engage the circuits necessary for extending the half-lives of happiness, pride, curiosity, and other positive emotions.

Attention Style and ADHD

There's an old Zen story: A student said to Master Ichu, "Please write for me something of great wisdom." Master Ichu picked up his brush and wrote one word: "Attention."

The student asked, "Is that all?"

The master wrote, "Attention. Attention."

The student became irritable. "That doesn't seem profound or subtle to me."

In response, Master Ichu wrote, "Attention. Attention. Attention."

In frustration, the student demanded, "What does this word *attention* mean?"

Master Ichu replied, "Attention means attention."

Very simple, very complicated; seemingly easy but sometimes maddeningly difficult. According to the *DSM*, ADHD comes in three varieties, marked predominantly by inattention, by hyperactivity/impulsivity, or by both equally. Inattention causes you to fail to focus on details and, as a consequence, to make careless mistakes in schoolwork, work, or other activities. It also causes you to have trouble organizing activities and makes you easily distracted. Hyperactivity is marked by fidgeting with your hands or feet, squirming in your seat, popping up when you are supposed to stay seated, and talking excessively. Impulsivity manifests itself as blurting out answers before questions have been finished, difficulty waiting your turn, and interrupting or intruding on others, as by butting into conversations or games.

The latest government data show that approximately 9.5 percent of the U.S. population ages four to seventeen—5.4 million children—have received a diagnosis of ADHD, and that number is rising. Between 2003 and 2007, the rate of ADHD increased by approximately 5.5 percent per year. While the precise cause of this dramatic increase is unknown, genetics alone clearly cannot explain it since Americans' DNA doesn't change remotely as fast as the rise in ADHD would require. Instead, the dramatic increase in incidence is likely due to either environmental factors or a broadening of the criteria used to diagnose ADHD.

While the symptoms of the different subtypes of ADHD suggest that several brain processes have gone awry, the core problem seems to be in circuits that underlie attention and "response inhibition," which reins in impulses. The ability to do so can be tested in the lab. In a typical experiment, children are shown a rapid series of pictures, such as faces. They have to press a button whenever they see an emotionally blank face but not when they see a face with an emotional expression. In an experiment with a hundred pictures, seventy are neutral and thirty are emotionally expressive, so the children should be pressing the button 70 percent of the time. Most people make errors, pressing the button when shown an emotional face, not because they cannot tell a blank face from an angry, happy, sad, or surprised one (that has been ruled out during a pretest) but because they cannot inhibit the tendency to press the button. Children and adults with ADHD make more such errors.

Brain imaging shows why. In an analysis of sixteen such studies involving a total of 184 people with ADHD and 186 normal controls, researchers at the New York University Child Study Center found that several regions of the prefrontal cortex important for selective attention and response inhibition were underactive in the ADHD group. In particular, the inferior prefrontal cortex, the brain's impulse-inhibiting center, seemed to be sitting this one out: While it lit up with activity in healthy controls, in kids and adults with ADHD it was sidelined. (As we will see in chapter 11, these are the brain regions that are strengthened by the forms of meditation that improve several aspects of attention.)

Another signature of attention is phase-locking, in which an external stimulus becomes synchronized with ongoing brain oscillations detected by electrodes on the scalp. Here, too, when this process goes awry, the result is ADHD: When scientists at the University of Toronto recently measured neural synchrony in nine adults with ADHD and ten healthy controls, they found much poorer synchrony in the ADHD group. Again, one of the key neural correlates of selective attention is dysfunctional in ADHD.

The point of such studies is not to amass more pretty pictures ("Look, this is your brain with ADHD"). At least, it shouldn't be. My hope, at least, is to use the results to pinpoint the neural activity that has gone off the rails and develop neurally based interventions to restore it to some semblance of normal. Today, the first-line treatment for ADHD is medication, notably, stimulants such as Ritalin that target neurotransmitters in the prefrontal cortex and thereby improve attention. The tendency of physicians to reach for the prescription pad is understandable: Most children who are treated for ADHD are seen by general practitioners who have neither the time nor the training to offer any other form of therapy. Specialists are in short supply, especially outside major metropolitan areas, and even psychologists and psychiatrists feel pressure (from insurers) to prescribe pills rather than to take the time to offer behavioral therapy.

But there are hints that alternatives to pills and all their side effects deserve further scrutiny. Although few studies have evaluated behavioral methods for training attention (no one, especially pharmaceutical companies, has a financial incentive to pay for them), those that have been done are promising. In one 2011 study from a team in the Netherlands, children with ADHD were given either attention training or perceptual training. For the latter, the eleven-year-olds honed their skills at seeing and hearing but without any attention component. For the attention training, they played a computer game in which they had to notice when enemy bots slipped into the scene and when their life force was dangerously low, and otherwise pay attention. After eight one-hour training sessions spread over four weeks, the children who received attention training—but not those who received perceptual training—showed significant gains on several objective measures of attention, including focusing despite distractions. The scientists did not do brain scans to identify any changes in neural activity that might explain the improved attention; that study is crying out to be done. But what we know so far provides hope that mental training can change the ADHD brain.

As I write this in 2011, an initiative at the National Institute of Mental Health (NIMH), a branch of the National Institutes of Health, is trying to take discoveries about the common underpinnings of different mental disorders and use them to better understand the brain bases of mental illness. The idea is that certain behaviors and psychological traits are common to multiple psychiatric disorders that, in today's taxonomy, are regarded as unrelated. For instance, low levels of Social Intuition—what I have labeled as the Puzzled end of that dimension—is a core characteristic of many people with autism. But it is also found in a number of anxiety disorders, particularly social phobia, and can occur in depression as well. Similarly, difficulty in sustaining positive emotion—in this scheme, having a Negative Outlook style—characterizes depression but is present in anxiety disorders as well as in schizophrenia. This suggests that treatments that are effective for one disorder may also be helpful for a disorder with which it shares a particular dimension of Emotional Style.

As things now stand, clinicians treat depression very differently than they do anxiety disorders and schizophrenia, and autism very differently than depression—in the medications as well as the psychological therapy they use. But NIMH recognizes that to make progress in understanding the brain basis of psychiatric disorder, which is crucial to treating the disorder, we have to tease out the dimensions of Emotional Style and identify their source in patterns of brain activity. That is precisely what I have tried to do with the six dimensions of Emotional Style.

This approach also promises to improve diagnoses of psychiatric disorders. In the traditional yes-or-no approach, someone who meets the minimum number of diagnostic criteria—six out of eleven possible symptoms of social anxiety disorder, for instance—has the disorder, and someone who falls short does not. As you can tell, the framework of Emotional Styles offers a very different perspective. While acknowledging the reality of mental illness, it shows that clear and unambiguous boundaries between normal and abnormal do not exist. A decision to transform your Emotional Style should therefore be based not on an arbitrary yes-no diagnosis but on your subjective appraisal of the kind of person you wish to be and the kind of life you hope to lead.

Just a few years ago, arguing that the dysfunctional brain activity underlying a mental illness could be treated with the power of the mind would have gotten you laughed out of the room (particularly one filled with psychiatrists or neuroscientists). But with the revolution in neuroplasticity, that possibility is, if not quite dogma, at least well within the mainstream. The power of the mind to change patterns of brain activity is the subject of the next chapter.

CHAPTER 8

■ ■ ■

The Plastic Brain

When I explain to audiences and classes that people have distinct Emotional Styles and that these styles reflect specific patterns of brain activity, they often leap to the conclusion that Emotional Style must therefore be fixed and, probably, genetically based. I hope that chapter 5 persuaded you that your Emotional Style is not a direct readout of the genes you inherited from your parents but is instead a complex mash-up of those genes plus the experiences you had as a child. Now I want to show you that the Emotional Style that saw you into adulthood does not need to be the one that describes you forever. Just because Emotional Style reflects patterns of brain activity—shaped by genes or not—doesn't mean that it is fixed, static, unchanging, and unchangeable. The reason is that the decades-old neuroscience dogma that the adult brain is essentially fixed in form and function is wrong.

Instead, the brain has a property called neuroplasticity, the ability to change its structure and patterns of activity in significant ways not only in childhood, which is not very surprising, but also in adulthood and throughout life. That change can come about as a result of experiences we have as well as of purely internal mental activity—our thoughts. Take experiences: The brains of people who have been blind from birth and who learn to read Braille, the writing system based on tiny raised dots that the fingers slide across, experience a measurable increase in the size and activity of areas in the motor cortex and somatosensory cortex that control movement and receive tactile sensation from the reading fingers. Even more dramatically, their visual cortex—which is supposedly hardwired to process signals from the eye and turn them into visual images—undertakes a radical career change and takes on the job of processing sensations from the fingers rather than input from the eyes.

Reading Braille is an example of an intense, repeated sensory and learning experience of the outside world. But the brain can also change in response to messages generated internally—in other words, our thoughts and intentions. These changes can increase or decrease the amount of cortical real estate devoted to specific functions; for example, when athletes engage in mental imagery, focusing on the precise sequence of movements required to execute, say, a forward two-and-a-half pike, the regions of the motor cortex that control the required muscles expand. Similarly, thought alone can increase or decrease activity in specific brain circuits that underlie psychological illness, as when cognitive-behavior therapy successfully quiets the overactivity in the "worry circuit," which causes obsessive-compulsion disorder. By mental activity alone, itself a product of the brain, we can intentionally change our own brain.

Hardwired Dogma

You wouldn't know about neuroplasticity from the ubiquitous drawings of the brain that label each of scores of regions with an authoritative-looking function—*this* spot in the motor cortex moves the left pinkie, *this* spot in the somatosensory cortex processes feeling from the right cheek. The idea that there is a one-to-one correspondence between structure and function dates back to 1861, when French anatomist Pierre Paul Broca announced that he had identified the brain region that produces speech: it is an area toward the back of the frontal lobes, he concluded from the autopsy of a man who had lost essentially all his powers of speech. (The discoverer got naming rights, and the brain's speech-producing region has since been known as Broca's area.)

With that discovery, scientists were off to the races, assigning particular functions to specific locations in the brain like a zealous zoning board. Thanks to German neurologist Korbinian Brodmann, whose studies of the brains of cadavers yielded structure-function relationships for fifty-two distinct regions, we got Brodmann areas number 1 (part of the somatosensory cortex, which processes tactile sensations from specific spots on the skin) through 52 (for the parainsular area, where the temporal lobe and insula meet). I have a soft spot for Brodmann 10, the front-most piece of prefrontal cortex, which has in creased most in size over the course of evolution and seems to allow us to multitask.

No region of the brain has been as precisely mapped as the somatosensory cortex. This strip of cortex runs roughly over the top of the brain from ear to ear; the left somatosensory cortex receives signals from the right side of the body, and the right somatosensory cortex receives signals from the left. But it's not one big, undifferentiated receiving area. Each part of the body is assigned a particular spot of the somatosensory cortex for processing. As a result, the somatosensory cortex is essentially a map of the body—but one that would give Google mappers a heart attack.

In experiments in the 1940s and 1950s, Canadian neurosurgeon Wilder Penfield found just how odd the map is. Penfield was performing brain surgeries, usually to treat epilepsy, but before the therapeutic part of each surgery he often took an exploratory detour. Using a mild electric shock, Penfield stimulated one spot after another on the exposed somatosensory cortex (the brain has no sensory receptors and so does not feel the little zaps), each time asking the conscious patient what he felt. The patients were shocked in the other sense of the term: When Penfield excited their somatosensory cortex, they felt that he had touched their cheek, or forehead, or arm, or leg, or other body part. In fact, all he had done was zap somatosensory neurons into firing. That firing was, to the patient, indistinguishable from the firing of the same neurons in response to an actual physical stimulus delivered to some part of the body. In this way, Penfield was able to "map" the somatosensory cortex, assigning each spot a corresponding part of the body.

And that's when he discovered that the cartographic anatomist apparently had a sense of humor. Although the hand is below the arm, the somatosensory cortex's hand—that is, the region that receives signals from the hand—abuts the region that receives signals from the face. The somatosensory representation of the genitals lies directly below the feet. The scale is off, too: The somatosensory representation of the lips dwarfs that of the torso and calves, while the hands and fingers are huge compared with the Lilliputian shoulders and back. The reason is that with more cortical space, a body part becomes more sensitive. The tip of your tongue, which has a large somatosensory representation, can feel the ridges of your front teeth, but the back of your hand, which has a small somatosensory representation, cannot.

As a result of the discoveries of Brodmann, Penfield, and others, for most of the twentieth century neuroscience held that these structure-function relationships are hardwired, a view encapsulated by the declaration of the great Spanish neuroanatomist Ramon y Cajal, who in 1913 called the adult brain "fixed, ended, immutable."

The belief in stasis carried over into the idea that particular patterns of activity must also be hardwired and, if not strictly unchangeable, at least persistent. According to this view, mental illnesses such as depression might be caused by underactivity in some areas of the prefrontal cortex and overactivity in the amygdala, and the underlying biology is as permanent as your fingerprints. Just to be clear, neuroscientists had recognized for decades that the adult brain can change at the cellular level to encode new facts and skills by strengthening connections between neurons. But this was change at the retail level, so to speak. Change at the wholesale level—making any alterations to the structure-function relationships depicted in those gorgeous brain maps—was thought to be impossible.

The Silver Spring Monkeys

Then the Silver Spring monkeys came along. These lab animals—rhesus macaques—were at the center of one of the most famous controversies in the history of biomedical research. Seventeen monkeys used in experiments at the Institute for Behavioral Research, in Silver Spring, Maryland, had gnawed off thirty-nine of their own fingers—a result, activists charged, of mistreatment and appalling living conditions. In fact, the main reason the monkeys had gnawed off their fingers was that they did not have any feeling in those fingers. The lab's lead scientist, Edward Taub, had surgically severed the sensory nerves leading from one or both arms in nine of the animals. (Convinced that his experiments would lead to effective new treatments for stroke, Taub wanted to see whether an animal needed sensory feedback in order to move a limb; the answer, he found, was no.) As a result, the animals lost all sensation in those limbs.

The case launched the animal rights movement in the United States. After the monkeys were rescued and spared any further research, they grew old in peace and eventually faced their final days. In a controversial move, scientists argued that since the remaining animals (several had died over the years of natural causes) were going to be euthanized to spare them further suffering, perhaps they could perform one final service to science: having their brains examined to determine what had happened as a result of some twelve years of having no sensations from their fingers, hands, or arms reach the somatosensory cortex.

The result of that sensory deprivation, a 1991 study showed, was stunning to a field of science that was still stuck in hardwired land. The region of the monkeys' somatosensory cortex that originally processed sensations from the fingers, hands, and arms had changed jobs: As a result of receiving no signals from those body parts for year after silent year, the region now processed signals from the face instead. Every bit of neuroscience wisdom said that a "deafferented region" of the brain—one deprived of signals from the part of the body it used to hear from regularly—would simply close up shop, for it was hardwired for that function and only that function. That's not what happened. The amount of brain now receiving sensations from the face had grown ten to fourteen square millimeters—"massive cortical reorganization," the scientists said, "an order of magnitude greater than those previously described."

Around the same time, other studies of monkeys—much more humane ones—were showing that the adult primate brain can change in response to something much less extreme and traumatic than amputation or nerve-cutting surgery: It can change in response to the way the animals live and behave. In one seminal study, scientists at the University of California, San Francisco (UCSF), trained owl monkeys to develop an extremely acute sense of touch in their fingers. In what was called the spinning disk experiment, they taught the monkeys to reach outside their cage to lightly place their fingers on a four-inch disk incised with wedge-shaped grooves. The idea was to let their fingers brush the disk, staying in contact with it as it spun, but without either stopping the spinning or getting thrown off like a kid who fails to hold tight to one of those old-fashioned playground merry-go-rounds. (You can get the same effect if you try to keep your fingers on a spinning LP record, trying to feel the grooves but making sure to neither stop the spinning nor let your fingers fly off.) Day in and day out, the monkeys underwent this exercise, until they had done it hundreds of times. Result: The region of their brain—specifically, in the somatosensory cortex—that received signals from the fingers that had been trained to feel the grooves in the spinning disk increased fourfold. Simply mastering a trick that required their fingertips to be extremely sensitive caused a region of the brain to expand into territory that used to have a different function (processing signals from other fingers). Structure-function relationships are not hardwired. Instead, the physical layout of the brain—how much space it assigns to which tasks and body parts—is shaped by how an animal behaves.

Just as the region of the brain responsible for feeling the sense of touch in a particular part of the body could change in response to experience, so could the region of the brain responsible for moving a part of the body. When scientists, also at UCSF, trained monkeys to tap a food pellet with sufficient dexterity to get it out of a tiny cup (one too small to accommodate more than a single monkey finger), they found a similar change in their brains: The region of the motor cortex responsible for moving the finger had doubled, taking over space that had previously controlled other parts of the body.

And what about human experiences? Might the brain changes discovered in monkeys pertain only to monkeys, while the human brain—arguably the most complicated structure in the universe, and one that you might think would be alterable at its owner's peril—is somehow protected against such tinkering? The place to look was in the brains of people with a very different sensory experience from the norm: those who are blind or deaf.

See the Thunder, Hear the Lightning

Perhaps you are not surprised that the fine structure of the somatosensory cortex and motor cortex—with the difference between a region that feels or moves a finger and a region that feels or moves a cheek measured in millimeters—can change in response to experience and behavior. But the brain is capable of even greater reorganization. Studies of the blind and deaf examined much larger, and arguably more fundamental, chunks of neural real estate: the visual cortex, which occupies nearly one-third of the brain's volume and is nestled toward the back; and the auditory cortex, which stretches across the top of the brain above the ears. You may be familiar with the folk wisdom that the blind have especially sharp hearing and the deaf have especially sharp eyesight, almost as if the gods were compensating them for their loss. In fact, blind people do not hear softer sounds, and deaf people cannot detect minimal contrasts or see in dimmer light than hearing people can. But there is indeed something to the idea of compensatory changes.

In people who are deaf from birth, objects in the peripheral vision are perceived not only in the visual cortex but also in the *auditory* cortex. Let me repeat that: The auditory cortex sees. It is as if the auditory cortex, tired of enforced inactivity as a result of receiving no signals from the ears, took upon itself a regimen of job retraining, so that it now processes visual signals. This rezoning has practical consequences: Deaf people are faster and more accurate at detecting the movement of objects in their peripheral vision than are hearing people.

Something comparable happens in people who are blind from birth or an early age. In them, of course, no signals reach the visual cortex, which as I mentioned is a huge chunk of the brain and, you'd think, one that Mother Nature would not allow to go to waste. She doesn't. In blind people who become proficient at reading Braille, the visual cortex switches jobs to processing tactile signals from these reading fingers. This discovery was so unexpected that some of neuroscience's most eminent practitioners refused to believe it, recommending that the journal *Science*, to which the discoverers had submitted it, reject the paper. Eventually, *Nature*, *Science*'s arch competitor, published it in April 1996.

The brains of the blind change in another way, too. When they use their peripheral hearing—to locate the source of a sound, for instance, something they tend to be better at than sighted people—they use their visual cortex. Their brains have undergone what we call compensatory reorganization, with the result that the visual cortex hears. Once again William James proved prescient. A century before these discoveries, in his 1892 book, *Psychology: The Briefer Course*, he wondered whether, if neurons got crossed inside the brain, "we should hear the lightning and see the thunder"—a foreshadowing of the profound functional alterations in the brain's primary sensory cortices that can result from experiences.

One final example of how extensive brain rewiring, even of regions as basic as the primary sensory regions, can be: Blind people use their visual cortex to remember words. Verbal memory is not even a primary sensory ability, yet when the visual cortex is not called on to perform its intended function, it can switch even to this higher-order cognitive function. (No such activation of the visual regions occurs when sighted people recall lists of words.) And in the blind, the visual cortex also generates verbs in response to nouns (like *throw* for *ball*). Again, it does not perform this function in sighted people. The ability of the visual cortex to process language came as a shock to neuroscientists.

To recap, the earliest hints that the brain can change, assigning a new function to a region that originally did something else, came from studies of lab animals and people who had been blind or deaf from birth. Skeptics could—and did—argue that these were aberrations, that the human brain is too complex and sophisticated to be this malleable, and that change in response to an extreme condition like congenital blindness or deafness does not imply change under normal circumstances. Just because young brains are highly plastic, able to rearrange things to compensate for the absence of sight or hearing, doesn't mean that normal adult brains can do so.

In chapter 1, I mentioned the cool "virtual piano player" experiment, in which Pascual-Leone and colleagues discovered that merely thinking about playing a keyboard exercise expanded the region of motor cortex devoted to moving the fingers. Pascual-Leone conducted another study that got to the heart of the objections about the normal adult brain's ability to change. He wondered whether the brain's primary sensory regions, supposedly as hardwired as hardwired can be, might in fact be malleable not only in people who are blind or deaf from birth, and in whom any such plasticity might be explained away as an aberration, but in sighted and hearing people, too.

Pascual-Leone therefore launched what he called the blindfold experiment. He and his colleagues recruited a group of healthy volunteers to spend five days in a safe environment at Beth Israel Deaconess Medical Center, in Boston, during which they were blindfolded 24-7. Before donning the blindfolds (which were equipped with photographic film along the bottom edge so that if a volunteer surreptitiously lifted the blindfold, the film would be exposed, ratting him out), the volunteers underwent fMRI scans to document their patterns of brain activity. Everything was as expected: When a volunteer looked at something, activity in his visual cortex increased, and when he heard or touched something, activity in his auditory cortex or somatosensory cortex, respectively, increased.

Then the volunteers spent five days blindfolded. To keep them from dying of boredom, the scientists had the volunteers spend their time in two sensorially intense activities: learning Braille and fine-tuning their hearing. Braille, as you recall, consists of patterns of raised dots that you run the tip of your "reading finger" (usually one or both of your index fingers) across, giving your fingertip an intense tactile workout. In the auditory task, the volunteers heard pairs of tones through headphones and had to indicate which was higher in pitch. That's pretty easy to do when one sounds like a baritone and one like a soprano, but harder when the tones are closer in frequency. At the end of five days of such exercises, with no visual input entering their eyes or their visual cortex, the volunteers underwent fMRI scans again.

This time, when the volunteers felt something with their fingers, activity in their visual cortex increased. When they heard something, activity in their visual cortex increased. The visual cortex is supposed to handle only sight, yet after a mere five days of an unusual sensory environment—no seeing but intense auditory and tactile stimulation—the supposedly hardwired visual cortex had switched professions, processing hearing and touching instead. This showed that such a radical change in function can occur not only in people who are blind from birth—in whom it might be dismissed as irrelevant to healthy brains, or as something that takes decades to develop—but also in people with normal sight, and in only five days. If the visual cortex, which seems like the most hardwired of all the brain's hardwired regions, can so quickly alter its function as a result of sensory input and sensory deprivation, surely it is time to question whether much about the brain really is fixed and unchangeable.

In all likelihood, the visual cortex did not grow new connections to the ears and fingers; five days wasn't time enough for that. Pascual-Leone suspects that instead "some rudimentary somatosensory and auditory connections to the visual cortex must already be present," left over from the period of brain development when neurons from the eyes and ears and fingers connect to many regions of the cortex rather than just the ones they're supposed to. When input from the retina to the visual cortex ceased because of the blindfold, the other sensory connections were unmasked. Even neuronal cables that receive no traffic for decades can start carrying signals again.

Neuroplasticity in the Clinic

The realization that sensory experience can rewire the brain has had important real-world consequences. The raid on the Silver Spring monkeys cost Edward Taub years of his life as he fought civil and criminal charges, but eventually he returned to research. Even as he was pilloried for his mistreatment of the monkeys, Taub insisted that everything he did was intended to help people who had been disabled by stroke. By the 1990s he had made good on his promise, tapping the power of neuroplasticity discovered in the Silver Spring monkeys—whose brain regions had been "remapped" to handle new jobs—to devise a therapy that has helped countless stroke patients function again. From the discovery that a region of the monkeys' brains could be trained to perform a new function, Taub inferred that people in whom a stroke had damaged one region of the brain could train a healthy region of their brain to assume the function of the damaged part.

He called the treatment constraint-induced movement therapy. I'll illustrate how it works with the example of someone in whom a stroke has disabled a region of the motor cortex, leaving one arm paralyzed. Taub would put this patient's good arm in a sling and her good hand in an oven mitt for about 90 percent of waking hours for fourteen straight days, so she could not use either, leaving her no choice but to try to use her paralyzed arm in the activities of daily living and the rehabilitation exercises he devised. Those exercises, six hours a day for two five-day weeks, involved intensive use of the "paralyzed" arm—which was actually slightly functional. The patient manipulated dominoes, held cards and cups and eating utensils, picked up sandwiches, and put pegs into holes—not well, not quickly, and often not successfully, at least at first. But after scores of hours of this, most patients made huge improvements and had regained most of the use of their "useless" arm and hand. They could dress themselves, feed themselves, and pick up objects, capably performing almost twice as many routines of daily living as stroke patients who did not receive constraint-induced movement therapy. And this improvement occurred not just in recent stroke victims. Even those who had suffered their stroke years before beginning therapy improved enormously, regaining their ability to brush their teeth, comb their hair, use a fork, drink from a glass, and the like.

Brain imaging revealed the reason for this success. Taub found what he called "a large use-dependent brain reorganization in which substantial new areas of the brain are recruited" to take over the function of regions that had been disabled by the stroke. "The area responsible for producing movements of the affected arm almost doubles in size, and parts of the brain that are not normally involved, areas adjacent to the infarct, are recruited," he said. This was the first time an experiment had demonstrated the rewiring of the brain as a result of physical therapy after a stroke.

As Taub's and other studies showed, this brain plasticity took any of three forms. In some patients, an adjacent region in the motor cortex assumed the function of the disabled region. In others, the premotor cortex, which usually only plans movements and does not actually order them executed, took over for the damaged region of the motor cortex. And in other patients, the brain reorganization was truly dramatic: If the stroke had disabled the right motor cortex (leaving the left arm paralyzed), then the corresponding region of the left motor cortex took over, yet with no apparent effect on its ability to do its original job of moving the right arm. In short, the brain has the power to re-cruit healthy neurons to perform the function of the damaged ones. Neuroplas-ticity enables the brain to reassign jobs.

The case for neuroplasticity was not quite airtight, however. Skeptics could still argue that it took place only under extreme conditions, such as a stroke. Taub would prove them wrong, too. He recruited violinists and other string musicians for a brain-imaging study, examining the region that controls the four fingers that dance across the strings to select notes. These "fingering digits" get an intense workout and must have superb fine motor skills—just like with the owl monkeys at UCSF who learned to gently rest their fingers on the spinning disk. And Taub discovered that his musicians were no different from the monkeys. In the violinists, the amount of space in the somatosensory cortex devoted to registering feelings from the digits of the left hand was much greater than that in nonmusicians, especially in those who began playing seriously before age twelve (though this expansion also occurred in people who took up the instrument as adults). Brains exposed to the demands of playing the violin undergo extensive alterations, displaying use-dependent cortical reorganization.

"Plasticity is an intrinsic property of the human brain," says Pascual-Leone. "The potential of the adult brain to 'reprogram' itself might be much greater than has previously been assumed," he and colleagues concluded in 2005. Neuroplasticity allows the brain to break the bonds of its own genome, which dictates that one region of the brain will "see" and another will "hear," that one spot on the somatosensory cortex will feel the right thumb and another the left elbow. This genetically guided blueprint is fine for most people under most conditions, but not all of us all the time—not when we lose our sight or suffer a stroke, not when we dedicate ourselves to mastering the violin. As a result, nature has endowed the human brain with a malleability and flexibility that lets it adapt to the demands of the world it finds itself in. The brain is neither immutable nor static but continuously remodeled by the lives we lead.

So far in our discussion of neuroplasticity, we have seen that the brain can change the function of particular structures in response to the sensory and motor demands placed on it. Intense motor training induces the brains of stroke patients to reorganize in a way that allows healthy regions to substitute for disabled ones; intense musical practice expands regions responsible for the sensitivity of the fingering digits; the absence of visual signals induces the visual cortex to process sounds or touch instead. In each case, the cause has been external to the brain—sensory or motor signals arriving with greater intensity (violinists, stroke patients in rehab) or not at all (the blind and the deaf). What about signals that come from the brain itself—that is, its own thoughts?

Mind over Matter

In chapter 1, I recounted the experiment in which merely thinking about performing a piano exercise expanded the region of the motor cortex responsible for moving those fingers. Let me tell you about two other fascinating experiments in which, to put it bluntly but accurately, the mind changes the brain.

Neuropsychiatrist Jeffrey Schwartz, of the University of California, Los Angeles (UCLA), had treated many patients with obsessive-compulsive disorder. In OCD, people experience upsetting, intrusive, unwanted thoughts, or obsessions, such as worrying that the stove is still on or believing that stepping on a sidewalk crack will trigger some calamity. As a result, they feel compelled to perform ritualistic behaviors, or compulsions, such as repeatedly running back home to check the stove or going to extremes to avoid stepping on a crack. Brain-imaging studies show that OCD is characterized by hyperactivity in two regions: the orbital frontal cortex, whose main job is to notice when something is amiss; and the striatum, which receives input from the orbital frontal cortex as well as the amygdala. Together, the orbital frontal cortex and striatum form what has been called the worry circuit, and in people with OCD it is buzzing with activity.

Rather than just drug his patients (antidepressants including Prozac, Paxil, and Zoloft helped some but usually not completely or forever), Schwartz got the idea of using a technique he employed in his own Buddhist meditation practice. Called mindfulness, or mindful awareness, it involves observing your thoughts and feelings from the perspective of a nonjudgmental third party. In *The Heart of Buddhist Meditation*, the German-born Buddhist monk Nyanaponika Thera described it as attending "just to the bare facts of a perception as presented either through the five physical senses or through the mind ... without reacting to them by deed, speech or by mental comment." In the case of his OCD patients, mindfulness meant learning to experience an OCD symptom without reacting emotionally, and learning to realize that the feeling that something is amiss is just the manifestation of overactivity in the OCD circuit. A patient would think, *My OCD circuit is producing another obsessive thought. I know it's not real but just static from a faulty circuit.* After many hours learning this technique, patients were better able to resist the OCD messages, reporting that their disease no longer controlled them. Neuroimaging also showed that activity in the orbital frontal cortex, the core of the OCD circuit, had fallen dramatically compared with what it had been before mindfulness-based therapy. Thinking about their thoughts in a new way had altered patterns of brain activity.

This finding is crucial to my belief that we can similarly alter the patterns of brain activity underlying Emotional Style, so let me offer one more example of how mental training can accomplish this. Clinical depression is character-ized by overactivity in specific regions of the frontal cortex, the seat of reason-ing, logic, analysis, and higher thought, in particular regions associated with anticipation—perhaps the cause of the endless rumination that grips people suffering from depression. There is, in addition, often underactivity in parts of the limbic system (the brain's emotion center) associated with reward and plea-sure. That would seem odd if you thought of depression as being marked primarily by an overwhelming sense of sadness, which presumably would show up as heightened activity in the limbic system. In fact, however, people with depression report that they experience what's called flat affect—an in-ability to experience soaring flights of joy, certainly, but also the absence of feelings such as curiosity or interest in the world.

Cognitive-behavior therapy, which was developed in the 1960s, is at bottom a form of mental training. It focuses on teaching patients to respond to their emotions, thoughts, and behaviors in a healthy way. The idea is to reappraise dysfunctional thinking, helping people escape the pattern in which they think, *The fact that she didn't want to go out with me a second time means I am a total loser and will never be loved.* Patients learn to recognize their habit of catastrophizing, of turning everyday setbacks into calamities, and with these cognitive skills, they can feel sadness and experience disappointment without tumbling into the abyss of depression.

Much as Schwartz taught his OCD patients to recognize obsessive thoughts and compulsions as the flotsam and jetsam of an overactive OCD circuit, so a group of pioneering psychologists taught patients with depression to regard depressive thoughts as simple electrical events in the brain. Scientists at the University of Toronto found that cognitive-behavior therapy has a powerful effect on the brain activity underlying depression. The therapy reduced activ-ity in the frontal cortex and raised activity in the limbic system. Patients ru-minated less and no longer felt emotionally dead inside. Their depression lifted, and in most cases it stayed lifted: Rates of relapse with cognitive-behavior therapy are much lower than with medication, which in any case seems to be no more effective than a placebo for anything but the most severe depression. But for our purposes, the bottom line is this: New patterns of thinking, learned through cognitive-behavior therapy, can alter brain activity in fundamental ways, enabling people to leave behind unhealthy patterns and go forward with new, healthier patterns that give them a renewed sense of joy and spare them the sadness, flat affect, and rumination that had proved so crippling.

In short, the revolution in neuroplasticity has shown that the brain can change as a result of two distinct inputs. It can change as a result of the experiences we have in the world—how we move and behave and what sensory signals arrive in our cortex. The brain can also change in response to purely mental activity, ranging from meditation to cognitive-behavior therapy, with the result that activity in specific circuits can increase or decrease.

In the next chapter, I will describe the beginning of my own journey of discovery about the power of the mind to change the brain.

CHAPTER 9

■ ■ ■

Coming Out of the Closet

I wouldn't say it was *the* reason I settled on Harvard as my graduate school (and you can be sure I didn't breathe a word of this to the admissions officers), but one of the school's attractions was the presence of another graduate student in psychology, Daniel Goleman. Dan would eventually become widely known as the psychology reporter at the *New York Times* and, later, as the author of the phenomenally successful book *Emotional Intelligence*, but in my senior year of college he caught my eye with a series of papers in an obscure publication called the *Journal of Transpersonal Psychology*. In 1971, he wrote a paper titled "Meditation As Metatherapy: Hypotheses Toward a Proposed Fifth State of Consciousness," and the next year he followed it up with "The Buddha on Meditation and States of Consciousness, Part 1: The Teaching" and "Part II: A Typology of Meditation Techniques." Neither meditation nor the Buddha were, needless to say, exactly in the mainstream of psychology research, so for a grad student at Harvard—where the psych department epitomized the mainstream, and where the hegemony of behaviorism made meditation about as welcome as a lecture on evolutionary biology at a creationism conference—to be writing scholarly papers about them was eye-catching, to say the least. I was looking forward to meeting Dan.

My very first class at Harvard, in the fall of 1972, was part of a course in psychophysiology, which met late in the day. I took a seat next to this scruffy-looking guy with a Jewish Afro and, on a hunch, turned and asked if he was Dan Goleman. He was, indeed. My question didn't come as a total surprise, since our mutual adviser, Gary Schwartz, had mentioned to Dan that I'd be starting grad school. After class, the last of the day for both of us, he asked if he could drive me home, so we walked to his car, a Volkswagen microbus. While it's a good bet that 99 percent of the other VW microbuses on college campuses in the early 1970s were decorated with pictures of the Doors, Jefferson Airplane, and/or Bob Dylan, Dan's was plastered from floor to ceiling with pictures of holy men from India! There were lamas on the doors, yogis on the visors, and maharishis on the seats. The whole thing felt like a rolling ashram.

Dan invited me back to his place, where we spent hours talking about how we had wound up at Harvard, about psychology, what each of us wanted to do with our lives, Dan's recent trip to India to study meditation, crazy yogis, and his unusual living situation: Dan was renting a room in the stately Cambridge mansion of David and Mary McClelland. It was my interview with David that clinched my decision to apply to Harvard for graduate school in the first place, so I was delighted to reencounter him. In chapter 2, I mentioned David's involvement in the Ram Dass affair and how Harvard had eventually fired Ram Dass. But by 1972 Ram Dass, apparently not holding a grudge, was living in the carriage house behind David's home. (He would go on to become a world-renowned spiritual teacher and author.) Mary, who had met David at a Quaker camp and married him in 1938, was a lovely, spiritual woman and a talented painter, keeping a studio in the basement.

For a kid from Brooklyn, entering the orbit of this (to say the least) interesting household was like stepping into a parallel universe, and the community at the McClellands' became an important source of alternative education for me as I went through graduate school. Let's just say that the goings-on there did not have a great deal in common with my day-to-day experiences at William James Hall. Many in the motley collection of household members, boarders, and general hangers-on dressed in handmade clothes they had brought back from India. The weekly meditation sessions were led by Ram Dass himself. The communal meals almost never included fewer than eight people. But what most attracted me to these people were their emotional styles! These were resilient, kind, positive people who seemed very socially tuned in and had remarkable equanimity. At a party celebrating their thirty-fifth wedding anniversary, the McClellands put on a slide show illustrating their life together. Susan and I—who had just started living together and had the usual trepidation about marriage—wondered how they had managed to pull it off. I asked Mary what it was like to be married for so long. Fixing us with her penetrating eyes, she declared, "Well, the first eighteen years were hell."

Since the McClellands and their circle credited their meditation practice for their remarkable combination of passion and serenity, that kindled in me an intense desire to try meditation myself and to become more than the dabbler I was (in college I had attended a few lectures about meditation and had taken yoga classes that included meditation, but that was it). Now that I had fallen in with Dan and the McClellands' household, I began meditating a few times a week—once with the group and the rest on my own. McClelland, a professor with an endowed chair at Harvard, had one foot very successfully planted in the world of academic psychology and one in the world of spiritual transcendence; I took his example as implicit permission to try the same.

To India

Toward the end of my second year of graduate school, I announced to my Harvard mentors that I wanted to take three months off to go to India and Sri Lanka to "study meditation." This was not met with universal enthusiasm. One professor asked why I wanted to waste three precious months of grad school on such nonsense, while another thought this would be the end of me as a budding scientist and that I would never come back. Luckily, it wasn't crucial that I get the department's blessing, but I did need to buy plane tickets and eat. This meant being as persuasive as I could possibly be with the National Science Foundation. The year before I had received a prestigious NSF graduate fellowship that paid for my tuition in full and also provided me with a then-princely stipend of a thousand dollars a month. How could I convince NSF to use this money in India and Sri Lanka? Apparently (since it worked), by arguing that I would study the relationship between meditation and attention, and between meditation and emotion. It was important for me to get firsthand experience of meditation in the cultures in which it had originated,

I argued. NSF said okay, and at the end of the spring semester—May 1974—off I flew to Asia. But not alone. I persuaded Susan, then a graduate student in psychology at the University of Massachusetts, Amherst (she subsequently went to medical school and became an obstetrician), to accompany me. The experience can't have been too much of a disaster: She married me in 1976, and we remain together to this day.

Our first stop was Sri Lanka, which was then called Ceylon. For a month and a half we stayed with Dan Goleman, his then-wife Anasuya, and their two-year-old, Govindass (yes, this was the heyday of Hindu influence on a certain slice of America) in a sprawling house they were renting in Kandy, in the hill country. Kandy was Ceylon's last royal capital and is known for its Buddhist Temple of the Tooth (one of the Buddhas is supposedly there) as well as other Buddhist and Hindu shrines. Dan and I rose early each morning, put on our sarongs and Harvard T-shirts, practiced meditation, and then spent hours working—which meant talking through how we might study meditation in a scientifically rigorous way. Afternoons were spent visiting monasteries to meet monks, most of whom belonged to the Theravada tradition of Buddhism, and just being (somewhat atypical) American tourists. The people of Kandy were remarkably welcoming to us, and we were often invited to dinner at the homes of those we had just met.

The only real shadow cast over this otherwise idyllic existence—and it was a big one—was the casual but brutal racism in the country. The Tamil minority were servants of the Sinhalese majority, but *racism* does not convey the contempt in which they were held. Having seen families' Tamil servants going to sleep for the night not in a bed but on the floor in a corner of the main room, I was not surprised when civil war broke out between these ethnic groups in 1983, killing tens of thousands of mostly innocent people before it finally ended in 2009 with the defeat of the Tamil rebel group by government forces.

In July 1974, Susan and I went to northern India, where we spent ten days in our first meditation retreat, at the former British hill station of Dalhousie. In those days traveling around India meant buses and, if you were lucky, trains (although luck extended only so far: the third-class cars, which were all we could afford, were teeming with chickens traveling with their owners). After an overnight train got us as far as Pathankot, we piled into a bus for Dalhousie. Did I mention that this was July? In India? We hadn't factored the monsoons into our plans, but nature had. As the bus wove through mountainous roads in a driving rain, suddenly what seemed like the entire side of the mountain beside us gave way. With a deafening roar boulders began raining down, a sea of tree-and-debris-filled mud washed over the road in front of us, and half the road itself slid down the mountainside. Then, silence, except for the pounding rain . . . and the percussive beats of my heart every time I peered over the precipice at the six-thousand-foot drop.

We sat there for the next six hours, grateful to be alive. We were almost as thankful that a bus eventually came from the direction of our destination—and got stuck on the *other* side of the washed-out road and pile of rubble. Since we were where they wanted to be, and they were where we wanted to be, the solution was obvious, if unappealing: Everyone in our bus clambered out into the driving rain, collected our stuff, carefully climbed over the rubble, and broad-jumped the gap in the road to the other side, while everyone on the other bus did the same. Now everyone was on the side of the washout they needed to be on, but the buses were not facing in the directions they now needed to go. We therefore had an interesting time navigating the hairpin turns and slick inclines backward (there wasn't room for the bus to turn around on the narrow mountain road and point itself in the direction of Dalhousie for several miles). Eventually, the bus managed a K-turn and, miraculously, we reached the retreat center a short time later.

Run by a very well-known Buddhist meditation teacher named Goenka, the center made up in the intensity of its meditation program what it lacked in creature comforts (there was no running water, and we slept in tents). The morning wake-up bell sounded at four thirty, the first meditation began at five, and all the retreatants—though obviously not the instructors—had taken a vow of silence. We would start with a one-hour sitting meditation and then switch to walking meditation, alternating the two for approximately fourteen hours a day, until ten at night, for the ten days of our stay. We would adjourn for two meals a day (no dinner) and for trips to the bathroom, but even then we would not break our silence. One day in August, a note was passed from one retreatant to another: President Nixon had resigned.

Goenka's instructions for our practice of vipassana (meditation designed to allow the practitioner "to see things as they really are") were very specific. We were to slowly and deliberately direct our attention to different parts of our bodies in turn—to what the tips of our noses were feeling, the different temperatures of air we inhaled and exhaled, how our leg bones felt against the floor . . . until we had completed a veritable *Gray's Anatomy* of vipassana. One goal of this form of meditation is to apprehend how your feelings and attitudes change. For instance, pain begins as pain. But as you focus on your bodily sensations, you begin to realize that what you thought was pain is just a concept, and if you can peer beyond the concept, you perceive a cluster of sensations—perhaps tingling in your feet, pressure in your knees, a burning in your calf muscles. The whole gestalt adds up to pain, but if you focus on its constituents, it's no longer painful—the sensations are still there, but the way we attend to them has changed. The new attitude is, "Oh, that's my feet tingling [or my knees burning]," but the mind learns not to conceptualize this galaxy of sensations as the aversive, unpleasant thing labeled "pain."

It will not surprise you to learn that this way of (not) reacting to pain does not come naturally. By the second day, Susan was muttering that she was ready to get the hell out of there and go back to Delhi, and (making an effort to keep her vow of silence) was going to write me a note to that effect. But first we went to Goenka's lecture that evening. "A lot of you are probably feeling a great deal of pain and would like to leave," he said, "but I'd like you to make a commitment to staying for just the next twenty-four hours." Susan, good sport that she is, hung in there (though she told me later that a main focus of her meditation was how we were going to get back down the mountain with the road washed out)—and after one more day everything changed. Just as Goenka had implicitly predicted, Susan mastered her attitude toward pain, adopting a nonjudgmental awareness of it: "Yes, my knees burn and my feet are tingling, but those are just discrete sensory experiences that I am not going to dignify or reify with the label 'pain.'"

Goenka taught that vipassana meditation offered a path to enlightenment and the eradication of suffering, but over the course of my hundred-plus hours of silent meditation I became convinced that it also had enormous, untapped potential for psychology and neuroscience. I had directly experienced a tectonic change in how I perceived the world, shaking off the concept of pain as if it were no more than a speck of lint on my shirt, and cultivating a deep and lasting sense of contentment in the moment. As a scientist, I had no doubt that what had occurred involved a change in my brain, presumably in the systems that govern attention and emotion.

Meditation Meets Science

Back at Harvard, in what was now the beginning of my third year in graduate school, I therefore began to do a little research on meditation. In one experiment, Dan Goleman and I studied fifty-eight people who had varying degrees of experience with meditation, from none at all to more than two years' worth. We administered some standard psychological questionnaires to them and found—drum roll, please—that more experience meditating was associated with less anxiety and greater attentional ability. We acknowledged that the difference might reflect different predispositions on the part of nonmeditators, novices, and experts—that is, that being able to focus and having little anxiety might enable someone to stick with meditation for two years, whereas being a neurotic, fidgety type would work against that. Without that acknowledgment, we would have seemed awfully naïve. Although I was thrilled that the paper was accepted by the *Journal of Abnormal Psychology,* publication was no guarantee of respect. When I told one of my professors about this work, he replied, "Richie, if you wish to have a successful career in science, this is not a very good way to begin."

The disdain of mainstream psychology was only one of the factors that made research on meditation less than desirable. The biggest impediment was that brain imaging had not been invented yet. The fairly crude EEGs that we used could detect electrical activity in regions of the cortex near the surface, where the electrodes were pasted, but no deeper. This meant that the vast majority of the living brain was opaque to science, including subcortical regions, which are so important for emotion. In the long run, though, not being able to study meditation scientifically in the 1970s turned out to be a blessing in disguise. It enabled me to turn my full attention to the study of emotion and the brain, which ultimately led to the development of affective neuroscience as we know it today. And by the time I was ready to study meditation, the neuroscientific tools were up to the task.

Although meditation would not be part of my scientific life for two more decades, it was very much a part of my personal life. I continued to practice daily, setting aside forty-five minutes each morning for what's called open-presence, or open-monitoring, meditation. A form of vipassana, it involves being fully aware of whatever is the dominant object in the mind at a given moment, whether a bodily sensation, an emotion, a thought, or an external stimulus, but without letting it take over your consciousness. I alternate open-presence with compassion or loving-kindness meditation, in which I begin with a focus on those closest to me, wishing that they be free from suffering, and then move out in an ever-expanding radius until that wish encompasses all of humankind. I have found this practice hugely beneficial. I live what most people would call a stressful, overscheduled life, typically putting in seventy hours of work each week; running a lab with dozens of graduate students, postdoctoral fellows, technicians, and assistants; raising millions of dollars from private and government funders to support everyone; vying for grants; and trying to stay at the top of a competitive scientific field. I believe my ability to juggle all this, with the small amount of equanimity I can muster, is a direct effect of my meditation practice.

I didn't make a habit of talking about meditation with my scientific colleagues, figuring that it was just enough outside the mainstream to be unlikely to help my very nascent career. But all this changed dramatically in 1992. In the spring of that year I screwed up my courage to write a letter to the Dalai Lama. I presumptuously asked the head of Tibetan Buddhism if it would be possible to study some of the expert meditators living in the hills around Dharamsala, to determine whether and how thousands of hours of meditation might change the brain's structure or function. I wasn't interested in measuring the patterns of brain activity that accompany meditation, though that might be perfectly interesting. Instead, I hoped to see how thousands and thousands of hours of meditation alter brain circuitry in a sufficiently enduring way as to be perceptible when the brain is not meditating. It would be like measuring the strength of the biceps of a bodybuilder when he's not doing curls: All that exercise enlarges the muscle, and you can measure that even when the bodybuilder is doing nothing more strenuous than lifting a latte. The yogis and lamas and monks living in the hills would be perfect for this, because they undertake meditation retreats lasting months or even years, which I suspected would have left a lasting impression on their brains. Of course, perfect for science was not necessarily perfect for the meditators. They had dedicated themselves to a life of solitary contemplation. Why would they ever agree to put up with the likes of me?

I got lucky. Although the Dalai Lama had been interested in science and engineering since he was a child, looking at the moon through a telescope in the palace at Lhasa and disassembling cuckoo clocks and watches, he had recently become interested in neuroscience in particular and was intrigued by what I had proposed. He wrote back, promising to reach out to the meditating hermits and lamas in the stone huts across the Himalayan foothills and request that they cooperate with my rudimentary experiment. This, obviously, was not easy. Neither mail nor phone nor carrier pigeon was an option, and since the closest meditator was holed up in a hut ninety minutes from the end of the nearest dirt road, the Dalai Lama couldn't exactly drop in and chat during his daily perambulations. Fortunately, however, the Dalai Lama had designated a monk on his staff to serve as liaison to the lamas and monks and hermits. This monk acted like a circuit rider in the nineteenth-century American West, visiting each meditator every few weeks to bring him food and make sure he was okay (many of the meditators were quite elderly). So in the spring and summer of 1992, this emissary of the Dalai Lama brought them something unexpected: a request from His Holiness to cooperate with some strange men who would be showing up in a few months to measure electrical activity in their heads. In the end, he persuaded ten of the sixty-seven meditators to indulge us.

This was not a one-man undertaking. Traveling with me to Dharamsala that November were Cliff Saron, whom you met in chapter 2 and who was by then a scientist at the University of Wisconsin with me, and Francisco Varela, a neuroscientist at Hôpital de la Salpêtrière in Paris. (Cliff had written such a persuasive grant proposal that we managed to wrangle $120,000 from a private foundation to support this study.) Also with us was Alan Wallace, a Buddhist scholar then at the University of California, Santa Barbara, who in 1980 had undertaken a five-month meditation retreat in these very hills after studying Tibetan Buddhism for ten years in India and Switzerland. Alan had been a student of the Dalai Lama in the early 1970s and received monastic ordination from him in 1975. We very much hoped that he would ease our acceptance by the meditators.

We all stayed in Kashmir Cottage, a guesthouse owned by the Dalai Lama's youngest brother, Tenzin Choegyal. T. C., as he is affectionately known, was not only our host but also our fixer, helping us figure out the protocols involved in meeting the Dalai Lama. In return, we turned one of his rooms into an electronics warehouse. This was back in the days when *computer* meant not a one-pound laptop but a suitcase-size box of electronics, and the other equipment we needed to carry out the study—electroencephalographs, lead-acid batteries, diesel generators, and video cameras—filled five steamer trunks. Gadget-loving T. C. was in heaven.

On the second morning of our stay, after a traditional Tibetan breakfast of eggs and tea, the four of us walked down the hill and across a plaza filled with begging children, lounging cows, and blankets spread with fruits and vegetables for sale to the Dalai Lama's residence. His sprawling compound was guarded by Indian soldiers carrying automatic rifles, and security was tight: We entered a two-room security shack, where we were called one by one for passport checks, bag X-rays, and hand pat-downs. Judged not to be risks, we exited security and began climbing a winding path that snaked past the dozen buildings in the compound—library, staff quarters, administrative buildings, audience halls, private quarters. Finally, we reached the anteroom, its hardwood walls and elegant bookcases giving it the feel of a little jewel box, where we waited to be summoned.

I was in a near panic. As I tried to formulate my opening words to the Dalai Lama, I was so nervous I couldn't come up with anything even remotely coherent. My heart was racing, I had broken into a cold sweat, and I was on the verge of a full-blown panic attack—at which point the Dalai Lama's chief of staff, a middle-aged Tibetan Buddhist monk dressed in the ubiquitous saffron robes, walked into the anteroom and announced that it was time.

He led us into the next room, which was furnished with a large couch for visitors, a spacious chair for the Dalai Lama, a smaller chair beside it for his translator, brightly colored Tibetan *thangkas* (embroidered silk scroll paintings) on the walls, and statues of Buddhist deities on the floor and shelves. I was the designated spokesperson for our group, but I was awash in self-doubt about what had possibly possessed me to think we might have anything at all to offer the Dalai Lama; I was sure we were wasting his time. But in the fifteen or twenty seconds it took for each of us to bow in greeting and introduce ourselves—eased by the fact that the Dalai Lama already knew Alan and Francisco—my terror and anxiety completely and utterly vanished. I felt instead a very deep sense of security and ease, suddenly confident that this was exactly where I needed to be. The words flowed out of me, and I heard myself proposing that he help us study the mental abilities and brain function of individuals who have spent years training their minds, to see whether or not mental training changes the brain.

Despite all he had to deal with, from the suffering of the Tibetan people to staying in the good graces of his Indian hosts, modernizing monastic education, and tending to his own spiritual practice, somehow the Dalai Lama had found time to get up to speed on neuroscience. He was intrigued by the possibility that Western science could learn something from the men who devote their lives to mental training in the tradition of Tibetan Buddhism, and he was actually grateful that there were serious Western scientists who wanted to take this on.

And that's why we—Cliff Saron, Alan Wallace, Francisco Varela, and I—found ourselves making like pack mules that first morning in Dharamsala in November 1992. When we set out from Kashmir Cottage, we hadn't quite worked out the logistics of lugging all this stuff into the hills where, as I said before, the closest meditator was a ninety-minute walk from the nearest road (actually, make that "road"). A Jeep took us that far, and we'd hired Sherpas to haul the seven backpacks we had stuffed with sixty pounds (each) of electronics and other gear, but as we gingerly picked our way up the mountain it occurred to me more than once that we were insane. The first time was when the "path" hugging the mountainside narrowed so much that I—who then weighed 140 pounds dripping wet—wished I were skinnier, the better to paste myself against the mountain and avoid plunging to my death two thousand feet below. The second was when the rocks blocking our path forced us to choose between over and around. "Over" required us to hoist ourselves over a five-foot-tall obstacle. "Around" meant placing one foot on this side of the boulder, holding on to it for dear life, reaching the other foot around to find a toehold on the other side, and praying that we could swing the rest of ourselves around to the other side rather than falling to a certain death. I don't know whether praying to every deity in the Buddhist pantheon helped, but we all survived.

Finally, up ahead we spied a stone hut. That's where we found a monk I will call by the standard honorific Rinpoche 1 (we promised them all anonymity), who had been living in mostly silent retreat for ten years. One of the most experienced meditators of the ten on the Dalai Lama's list, Rinpoche 1 was in his sixties and in failing health and did not exactly embrace our mission. (Alan Wallace, whom Rinpoche 1 remembered from the months he had spent in retreat among them, translated our English into Tibetan and the lamas' responses into English.) At this point we simply wanted to establish a relationship, explain our goal, and demonstrate which experiments we hoped to do. One was the Stroop test, in which the word for a color is written in ink of a different color, such as *blue* printed in red, and the task is to read the word without being distracted by the ink color. It is a test of concentration, of the ability to screen out distraction. But Rinpoche 1 explained all too modestly that his own meditation practice was mediocre at best (something he attributed to a gallbladder problem), and that if we wanted to learn the effects of meditation, why, we should just meditate ourselves! We had failed to take into account the fact that humility is a core value of Tibetan Buddhism, and even describing one's meditation might be construed as boastful. We left Rinpoche 1's hut without so much as an interview, let alone any EEG data.

We didn't do much better with Rinpoche 2, even though he had been one of Alan Wallace's teachers. In this case, the problem was other scientists. Rinpoche 2 told us about a renowned yogi named Lobzang Tenzin, also from the hills above Dharamsala, who had traveled to Harvard Medical School for what scientists there promised would be noninvasive studies of meditation. But the Harvard researchers had drawn Lobzang's blood—and three months after his return to Dharamsala he was dead. Rinpoche 2 was certain the scientists' meddling had killed his friend. And another thing, he told us over the course of what became a three-hour debate: It makes no sense to try to measure the mind, which is formless and nonphysical. If we did succeed in measuring anything, he assured us, it would be completely unimportant in terms of understanding the effects of meditation.

This is how it went through monks three, four . . . through ten. One kindly advised us to pray to the Dalai Lama for success in our work. Another suggested we return in two years, by which time he might have achieved some modest success in attaining *shamatha*, a Sanskrit word best translated as "meditative quiescence," whose goal is to block out distractions so the mind can focus on an object with clarity and stability. Others feared that undergoing our weird tests would disrupt their meditation practice. But the most consistent theme was that expressed by Rinpoche 2: Physical measurements were simply inadequate for discerning the effects of meditation on the mind. Use EEG to detect, say, the compassion that meditation has the power to cultivate? Please. By the time we reached our last monk, we were 0 for 10.

Despite the scientific failure, I felt we had succeeded on another level. One of the monks had been held for many years and tortured in a Chinese prison in Tibet, finally escaping to Dharamsala. He described to us in haunting detail the moment-by-moment changes he had experienced as a result of compassion meditation, which he practiced regularly during his captivity. The sadness and despair and anger that initially filled his mind, he explained to us, gave way, a little more each day, to a feeling of compassion, including for his captors, whom he began to view as suffering from an affliction of the mind not of their own doing and so, in a sense, as being fellow sufferers. Surely, I felt, this extraordinary capacity could teach us something about the mind and the brain.

After ten days of trekking into the hills, we finally gave up on the idea of collecting scientific data on the meditators. Before leaving Dharamsala, however, we had another audience with the Dalai Lama, telling him that our hopes of collecting the first data on the neurological effects of long-term meditation had come to naught. We explained the reasons the adepts had declined our entreaties, their suspicion of our machines, and the worrisome accounts of what had happened to other monks who cooperated with Western scientists. As the Dalai Lama sat listening to our sorry tale, he suddenly burst out, "What if you tried again with long-term practitioners—but only those who have traveled in the West and are more familiar with Western thinking and technology?" None of the meditators in the hills had had extensive contact with the West or with science. But someone who had wouldn't suspect that electrodes might disrupt their meditation practice. Maybe we could invite such monks to laboratories in the West, rather than trying to test them in the field, and thus make use of the controlled environment there. (Bonus: no more trekking up mountains with hundreds of pounds of equipment!) I was instantly intrigued. And when the Dalai Lama promised to put in a good word for us with some of the Buddhist adepts in his circle, I knew we were in.

But he had a request of his own. He understood, he told us, that psychology research focused almost exclusively on negative emotions—anxiety, depression, fear, and sadness. Why, he asked, couldn't scientists instead harness the tools of modern neurobiology to study virtuous qualities such as kindness and compassion? I didn't know quite how to respond. I stammered something about how most biomedical research in the West is driven by a desire to treat disease, and that this model was imported into research on emotions: Since anxiety and depression and the like are problems and even illnesses, they command the lion's share of scientific attention, whereas since love and kindness are not problems, they are largely ignored. But even as I explained this, it rang hollow to my own ears. Surely, the more we knew about positive emotions, the better chance we would have to train people to cultivate them. Yet (as I learned when I got back home), the term *compassion* was not even listed in the index of any major psychology textbook in those days. I vowed then and there to do what I could to remedy this. I would do everything in my power, I told the Dalai Lama, to put compassion on the scientific map. I also vowed to be more open about my interest in meditation, to finally come out of the closet with my professional colleagues about my own meditation practice. By this time I was a full professor at the University of Wisconsin and had won several professional awards. What did I have to lose?

Monks in the Lab

Back in Madison, I dove into research on the neural basis of Emotional Style, emotion regulation, and individual differences in emotional reactivity, but I also laid the groundwork for rigorous studies of meditation. If you read the accounts of scientific research in the press, you're likely to get the idea that a researcher thinks of an interesting question, recruits human volunteers to study, and then after a little while has fascinating results. If only. First of all, simply getting permission from your university to do research on people—and I'm not talking about invasive surgery or experimental drugs but simply having people fill out questionnaires—is so laborious and time consuming that some labs have a full-time staffer who does nothing but fill out the paperwork and get research proposals through this process. In addition, once the details of an experimental design are settled (which can take a lot of time), a new experiment always requires computer programming, which can take months, and any new protocol requires extensive pilot testing in which a few participants are put through all the tasks—again, a months-long undertaking.

The first payoff from the Dalai Lama's promise to put in a good word for us with expert meditators came in 2001, when one of the most extraordinary human beings I have ever known walked into my lab. Matthieu Ricard, who was born in France in 1946, had been a Tibetan Buddhist monk since 1967, but he took a somewhat circuitous path to that calling. Matthieu is the son of the renowned French philosopher Jean-François Revel and the abstract painter Yahne Le Toumelin, so he grew up amid the incredible intellectual ferment that was postwar Paris. In 1972 Matthieu received a Ph.D. in molecular biology from the Pasteur Institute, where he worked with Nobel laureate François Jacob, and that same year he decided to forgo a conventional life in science and instead moved to the Himalayas, where he trained to become a Buddhist monk.

Matthieu was therefore key to bridging the chasm between the ancient traditions of Tibetan Buddhism and modern science: He understands the need for a control group and how to do a linear regression but is also an adept meditator. He first lent his brain to science when he allowed Francisco Varela, one of my co-sufferers during the "study" of the long-term meditators around Dharamsala, to take measurements of his brain activity while he meditated, but the work was never published. So when the Dalai Lama put out the word to expert meditators who were comfortable with the West and/or science to participate in such experiments, Matthieu (who spent a good deal of time with the Dalai Lama, serving as his translator during trips to Europe) was the first to enlist.

Matthieu came to Madison in May 2001. We knew we wanted to measure brain activity during meditation, probably with fMRI, but it wasn't that straightforward. Those colorful brain scans that so delight the public ("Here is your brain on Tetris") bear about as much resemblance to the actual data as a Rembrandt does to a palette covered in paint smears. First of all, the raw data are digital readouts; the reds and blues and other hues you see on particular regions of the brain are arbitrary colors. More important, fMRIs do not measure brain activity in isolation; everything they produce is the result of subtracting the activity that characterizes the brain at rest, or in some baseline state, from the activity during the task you're interested in, be it moving a finger or forming a mental image of Angelina Jolie. That means the baseline state is crucial; you don't want it to include anything that overlaps with the activity of interest if that overlap is an important component of the activity. For instance, if you are interested in the neural activity that produces visual imagery, you do not want your participants to watch something external as a baseline, because the brain uses some of the same machinery to form a visual image in the mind's eye as it does to perceive something real in the outside world. What could we use for the baseline, or control condition, to subtract from the meditation condition?

Another issue was how long Matthieu would have to meditate before being "in a meditative state." Entering a meditative state is not like throwing a switch. We'd have to give Matthieu time to get there and to hold it long enough to truly feel he was in a meditative state. That was something Matthieu himself would judge. The literal translation of the Sanskrit word for *meditation* is "familiarize," meaning that the adept is familiar with his own mind. Just as an oenophile tasting a familiar Syrah can recognize it instantly, so an experienced practitioner recognizes when he is in a meditative state. However, if we waited too long to begin collecting fMRI data or let the meditation go on too long, we might tax Matthieu's ability to remain motionless in the very uncomfortable MRI tube. From a research perspective, the ideal would be short periods of meditation alternating with short baseline periods.

After some trial and error, Matthieu decided that two and a half minutes was the right amount of time for each meditation session. For the baseline condition, he suggested a state called *lung ma bstan* (pronounced *lung ma ten*), a Tibetan expression that describes a mental state in which you are not sleeping or meditating but are not particularly attentive to anything, either. Matthieu said it was a state characterized by not trying to do any particular task and not being disturbed by any strong emotions or thoughts—a state of neutral indifference. For the meditation condition, he proposed that he alternate compassion meditation with open-presence meditation and devotion meditation (in which the meditator visualizes one of his most important spiritual teachers and focuses on the powerful feelings of respect, gratitude, and devotion he feels for him). Our programmers stayed up all that night writing the computer code that controls the data collection in the MRI, in this case so that the data stream would be marked with each change in mental state, such as from compassion meditation to baseline, and also controls when different stimuli are projected onto the video screen inside the tunnel. The timing script is crucial, since when we read the raw data, we needed to be able to say, "Ah, here is when Matthieu switched from lung ma bstan to devotion meditation."

Of course, the whole thing crashed as soon as we started early the next morning. No sooner had Matthieu slid into the MRI tube, donned the headphones through which we would communicate with him from the control room, and adjusted the fiber-optic goggles through which we would project visual instructions than the software crashed and scanning ceased. We peered through the window into the MRI room to make sure Matthieu looked comfortable, then got on the intercom and explained to him that we needed to fix something in the software and to please wait. The code had to be rewritten on the fly while Matthieu waited patiently.

When we were finally ready to try again, I read my script: "Okay, Matthieu, lung ma bstan." Wait three minutes. "Matthieu, now please compassion meditation." Wait two and a half minutes. "Now lung ma bstan." After six cycles of this, Matthieu took a short break, and then we switched to focused attention. Matthieu concentrated on a dot displayed on a video screen inside the MRI tube, again alternating with lung ma bstan. Then six cycles of open-presence meditation, in which Matthieu expanded his field of focus until it encompassed an entire panorama, as if surveying the world from fifty thousand feet up. Finally, six cycles of devotion meditation. It was a marathon session, lasting from seven in the morning until one in the afternoon. At the end of what would have left most volunteers as limp as a dishrag (and about as energetic), Matthieu emerged from the MRI tube for the final time with a beatific smile on his face and wanting to know only one thing: Did we get what we needed?

Usually there is no great rush to process and analyze MRI recordings, but this was no ordinary session. The Dalai Lama was going to show up on my doorstep the next morning.

When I was in Dharamsala in April 2000 for one of the periodic meetings between the Dalai Lama and Western scientists, organized by the Mind and Life Institute, he peppered me with questions about how specific methods to investigate the brain were used and what they allowed us to infer about brain function. How did EEGs work? How quickly did they change? What about fMRI and PET—what did they do better? At that time, the University of Wisconsin was building a major new brain-imaging lab, now called the Waisman Laboratory for Brain Imaging and Behavior, which I direct. Answering the Dalai Lama as best I could, I finally blurted out, "Your Holiness, I would love for you to visit my laboratory so I can show you exactly how these measurements are made." It took only three minutes of consultations to set a date with his somewhat taken-aback assistants (after all, the Dalai Lama is not only the spiritual leader of the world's 2.5 million Tibetan Buddhists, but was at that time also the head of the Tibetan government in exile, and as such his calendar was packed with everything from spiritual teachings to meetings in the White House): He would visit my lab the following May.

Suddenly, May was here.

After Matthieu's session, I therefore had a team of three graduate students and postdocs pull an all-nighter to analyze the data. I very much wanted to have the first findings on long-term practitioners—well, on one long-term practitioner—ready to present to the Dalai Lama the next morning. I raced down to the lab at six thirty, my heart in my throat as I waited to learn whether we had gotten anything useful. I met my exhausted research team as they were gulping down strong coffee from our new espresso machine; we were all running on adrenaline and caffeine, feeling we had arrived at a historic moment in the meeting of East and West, Buddhism and science, monks and fMRIs. And what we saw in Matthieu's data were the first impressions that engaging in specific forms of meditation evokes dramatic changes in brain function that our tools could measure. We all sat down in front of several computer monitors. The students and postdocs pulled up structural images of Matthieu's brain, on which were superimposed blobs of color that represented different degrees of activation throughout the entire brain for each meditation condition compared with lung ma bstan. I wanted to see compassion, focused attention, open-presence, and devotion side by side. With my mind racing and heart pounding at this first glimpse into a meditating brain, I was struck by differences among the four types of meditation. Although the distinctions between these conditions were purely mental—Matthieu was merely thinking different thoughts—the brain images showed clear differences in activity patterns. I had a strong sense that we had just crossed a threshold and that history was being made.

After assuring myself that the sessions with Matthieu had not been a total bust, I dashed upstairs to greet the Dalai Lama, whose arrival had all the trappings of a state visit. He travels with an entourage of staffers, translators (although his English is pretty good), and, as a visiting head of state, Secret Service protection. So it was a somewhat unwieldy group that trudged through the hallways and squeezed into labs, but the Dalai Lama was enthralled, even before we got to anything that had to do with neuroscience. I could barely get him out of the machine shop, where technicians use a drill press, precision saws, metalworking equipment, lathes, and vises to manufacture apparatuses we need but can't buy off the shelf. The Dalai Lama likes to say that if the whole reincarnation-of-the-thirteenth-Dalai-Lama thing (in which he was identified, at age two, as the successor to the previous head of Tibetan Buddhism) hadn't happened, he would have been an engineer. As a child in the palace at Lhasa, he loved taking apart car headlights, for example, and has never lost his love of gadgets. The drill press was a big hit.

When I finally managed to herd everyone into the MRI room, I had my fingers crossed that my usually reliable parlor trick would work. One of my students slid into the MRI tube as the Dalai Lama and I watched from the control room. After the equipment was turned on, I waited a minute while the student lay still and then asked him to move the fingers of his right hand. Presto: After some quick data processing, the motor cortex lit up (this works virtually 100 percent of the time, which is why I always use it to demonstrate how an fMRI captures brain activity). The Dalai Lama, however, wasn't done. He asked me if I could ask the student to just *think* of moving his fingers. No problem: The motor cortex again became active, although less so than during the actual finger movement. The Dalai Lama was delighted that something as purely mental as an intention or visualization produced brain activity so similar to something more physical—that is, finger movement.

We then drove to the Fluno Center, an executive conference center owned by the university, where the Dalai Lama was staying, for a meeting on the latest scientific findings on meditation. This is where I wanted to tell him about our experiment with Matthieu. I projected the images that had just been processed a few hours ago on a large screen in front of us. Since Matthieu was our only subject, I warned the Dalai Lama, we couldn't give too much credence to what we found, but it certainly looked as if something different was happening in the brain during the four meditative states than in the baseline state.

During compassion, both the insula and motor cortex were highly activated. During focused attention, the classical network of attention areas, including the prefrontal and parietal cortices, were activated. During open-presence, there was widespread activation of many brain regions. During devotion, we saw strong activation in the visual cortex, presumably as Matthieu visualized his teacher.

The Dalai Lama wanted to be sure: There was no change in external stimuli, right? This reflected purely mental activity, like the student who only *thought* about moving his fingers? Yes, I assured him—all the while torn between thinking that this was very cool and knowing that it wasn't science, at least not yet. It was only one subject during one run, and the whole thing could be garbage. Science is a long, laborious, even tedious process, I warned; we weren't going to announce any findings to the world until we had rigorous data from many, many meditators. And—although I kept this part to myself—it wasn't that surprising that meditation produces distinct patterns of brain activity. That goes without saying—anything the mind and therefore the brain does is marked by specific patterns of neuronal firing in specific areas, just as your muscles have particular patterns of electrical activity when you work out.

The Dalai Lama saw more clearly than we could that the field of contemplative neuroscience had just been born. Although he understood that it would take years until we had enough data to draw conclusions about how meditation not only produces distinct patterns of brain activity in real time but also leaves enduring changes in that activity—so that the brain of a meditator is different from that of a nonmeditator even when she is not meditating—he thought the research had the potential to transform humanity. Mental training might have the power to cultivate positive qualities of mind, as Buddhists have long taught as well as experienced, and to relieve great suffering, increasing the world's store of compassion and loving-kindness. But ours is a scientific age, the Dalai Lama knew. It would take more than the testimony of Buddhists to persuade people of the potential of mental training. It would take science.

Years later, I would look back on this day through a lens provided by Nobel laureate Francis Crick, the codiscoverer of the structure of DNA, who wrote this about new hybrid scientific fields:

"In nature hybrid species are usually sterile, but in science the reverse is often true. Hybrid subjects are often astonishingly fertile, whereas if a scientific discipline remains too pure it wilts."

Remaining too pure was not going to be a problem. I had committed myself to using the tools of modern Western science to illuminate phenomena and investigate methods of mental training that have formed the core of Buddhist teachings for twenty-five hundred years. By bringing together two approaches to understanding the nature of reality, I hoped, perhaps we would get a more complete and unbiased picture of the human mind. Now I had to hope that bringing together the two worlds would indeed yield Crick's hybrid vigor and not a sterile cross.

In the next chapter, I will describe the beginning of my own journey of discovery about the power of the mind to change the brain.

CHAPTER 10

■ ■ ■

The Monk in the Machine

Hard on the heels of our "triumph" in the hills of Dharamsala—that would be the "study" in which not a single one of the monks we approached agreed to participate—I realized that doing research on long-term meditation practitioners had a few drawbacks; the difficulty of obtaining cooperation was only one of them. More fundamental was the fact that people who dedicate their lives to spirituality and mental training, racking up thousands and thousands of hours of shamatha or vipassana or other forms of meditation, may not be typical of humankind, to put it mildly. Very few of us elect to spend such large blocks of time in silent mental training and contemplation. Even if I did eventually discover that the patterns of activity in the brains of long-term meditators are markedly different from the patterns in novice meditators or nonmeditators (which I indeed did, as I will describe later), that might not mean what it seems at first sight: Maybe the reason the brains of long-term meditators differ from those of other mortals is that they were born that way. Maybe that congenital brain difference causes someone to choose a contemplative life in the first place. Maybe the brain difference is not the *result* of meditation but the cause. Since we didn't have data on what the monks' brains were like before they took up meditation, we couldn't rule that out.

This realization was only one reason I put plans to study long-term meditators on hold. Another was that people roll their eyes when they hear how many hours "long term" actually means: upwards of ten thousand. Or, as a back-of-the-envelope calculation shows, two hours a day for seven days a week for 714 weeks—nearly fourteen years. Do you have time for only one hour a day rather than two? Then you're looking at twenty-eight years. You can do the rest of the math, but the implication is clear: Most people with families, jobs, and other claims on their time (like sleeping and eating) know they will never meditate that much in their lives.

These concerns—that long-term meditators might start with unusual brains, and ten thousand hours of meditation is beyond the reach of most people—pointed to one solution: Rather than compare meditators to non-meditators, I would study the effects of shorter-term meditation and track people over time to see if their brains changed.

Mindfulness-Based Stress Reduction

My chance to do a longitudinal study of meditation came in 1999. At the time I was a member of a research network on mind-body interactions established by the MacArthur Foundation (better known for awarding "genius grants"), an interdisciplinary group of about a dozen scientists and scholars who met half a dozen times a year to think up outside-the-box research that traditional funders were unlikely to touch. Although I had received funding from the National Institute of Mental Health continuously since 1978, I knew that applying for a grant to study meditation would be a waste of time. Over the course of one three-day meeting we tossed around the idea of studying mindfulness-based stress reduction (MBSR), and MacArthur generously gave us about $250,000 to do it.

MBSR is the most widely taught secular form of meditation in academic medical centers throughout North America and Europe. Developed by Jon Kabat-Zinn, of the University of Massachusetts Medical School in Worcester, the eight-week course teaches people to engage in mindfulness, the form of meditation in which you practice nonjudgmental, moment-to-moment awareness. Let me take the three parts of that description in reverse order. By "awareness," I mean that while sitting in a quiet place, you focus on whatever sensations your body is experiencing or whatever thoughts and emotions your mind is generating. You might start by feeling the pressure of the chair. Or the tension in your legs. Or how your elbow feels compared with your shoulder. Then you might move on to notice that as you take mental inventory of your physical sensations, a thought about what to make for lunch pops into your mind. Or you notice that your brain feels suddenly quiet. The "moment-to-moment" part describes how you take each sensation or thought as it comes. Finally, the "nonjudgmental" part is key. If your legs feel tense, you do not scold yourself for having difficulty relaxing; your reaction is closer to "Huh, tense legs; interesting." Similarly, for any thoughts and emotions, you do not intentionally pursue a thought as you ordinarily might (*Hmmm, lunch. I need to buy more mayo. Maybe I should have just a salad. I really need to eat less. Why am I thinking about this when I should be meditating? I'll never get this.*). If those thoughts arise, you observe them disinterestedly, as if from the perspective of a dispassionate observer, but do not take them to heart. They're just the interesting exudations of your brain's synapses and action potentials.

By now, in 2011, dozens of clinical trials have shown that MBSR can relieve psychological distress in breast cancer survivors, reduce side effects in organ-transplant recipients, relieve anxiety and depression in people with social anxiety disorder, and help people cope with chronic pain. In 1999, however, there had been no randomized controlled studies of MBSR, and little was known about its biological effects. We meant to change that.

We therefore contacted Promega, a biotech company just outside Madison, whose CEO, Bill Linton, is a UW alumnus and member of some university advisory boards. At one university function he and I got to talking about my work, and he opened up about how interested he was in meditation and in questions about the nature of consciousness and how it arises. This man, I thought, might actually be receptive to my doing a crazy study on his employees. So I made my pitch: Could my colleagues and I come to his offices and teach his employees mindfulness meditation and then assess how it had affected some measures of health as well as mental function?

Bill was enthusiastic. He made the company e-mail list available to us, and we used it to advertise for volunteers. We held four information sessions over the course of a month, in which I explained that some of the volunteers would learn a technique of stress reduction that was derived from Buddhist meditation, and some would be placed in a "wait-list" control group, which meant undergoing the same assessments as their coworkers learning stress reduction but not actually taking the classes. Which group someone wound up in would be totally random. After the study was over, though, people in the wait-list control group would be given the opportunity to learn MBSR. The reason we needed this kind of control group, we explained, was to ensure that people learning MBSR and people not learning it had the same interest in the class and a comparable motivation to take it. If we just accepted volunteers for MBSR, we'd be back to the problem with long-term meditators: We wouldn't be able to rule out the possibility that people opting to learn meditation might be different from the outset from people who chose to sit it out. We eventually got forty-eight volunteers, enough to proceed. Now it was up to Jon.

When I first met Jon Kabat-Zinn, in 1973, he had just accepted a position at UMass to develop a stress reduction program. That was not exactly the typical career path for someone who had just received a Ph.D. in molecular biology from the Massachusetts Institute of Technology, as Jon had, but even then he knew he wanted to devote himself to extracting what he had learned from his own meditation practice and presenting it in a way that an ordinary person who had never had any contact with the meditation disciplines could understand. Not surprisingly, when I told Jon about the study I was launching, he was not only thrilled to participate but he wanted to teach the MBSR course himself. This would be the first truly randomized controlled trial of MBSR, and Jon wanted to be present at the creation.

Now, the logistics for this were not trivial. Jon would not only teach the course—one two-and-a-half-hour session each week for eight weeks—but would also interview each prospective participant prior to the course and participate in the debriefing afterward. Oh, and after the sixth class, there would be an all-day retreat. Suffice it to say that Jon accumulated an impressive number of frequent-flier miles as he commuted weekly to Madison for ten straight weeks. Even getting stuck overnight in Chicago didn't faze him.

Before the first class, in September 1999, we gathered baseline data on all the volunteers. We measured brain electrical activity with EEG, focusing on the prefrontal cortex because that's where left-right asymmetry is associated with positive or negative emotions and greater or lesser Resilience. We also administered questionnaires that assessed how much anxiety and stress people felt, by asking them whether they agreed or disagreed with statements such as "I worry too much over trivial things" and "I often have disturbing thoughts."

Then the participants assigned to the class began learning MBSR—nonjudgmental, moment-to-moment awareness. Jon started them off with mindfulness of breathing, in which you focus on your breath: in and out, slower or faster, feel the air flowing through your nasal passages.... Then he moved on to mindfulness of the body: Lie on your back and, slowly and calmly, notice the sensations in different parts of your body; feel the floor against your shoulder blades and elbows; feel your feet splaying out as they relax; feel the tingle in your ankles.... Jon next had each participant eat a single raisin, taking five minutes to do so, noticing all the sensations as they chewed and savored and, finally, swallowed. He taught them mindful yoga, in which you go through simple poses (such as downward dog, in which you form an inverted V with your body, your hands outstretched on the floor and your rear end up in the air) in order to bring about increased awareness of bodily sensations. In later sessions Jon also read poetry to the class, choosing poems that capture some of the mental qualities at the core of mindfulness (the works of Rumi, the thirteenth-century Persian and Sufi mystic, were perfect for this). After the sixth class we held an all-day retreat one Saturday, which allowed Jon to take the participants through more intensive periods of practice as well as long, silent mindfulness meditation.

I have described the training in some detail to show that although eight weeks seems trivial compared with the thousands of hours a long-term meditator accumulates, it was fairly intense—intense enough, I hoped, to cause some measurable, significant changes in Emotional Style. In particular, we were interested in the Resilience and Outlook dimensions.

The classes ended around Thanksgiving, which happens to coincide with the onset of flu season. We took advantage of this by giving everyone—class takers and the control group—a flu shot, for reasons I'll explain below. We also repeated all the measurements we had made at the start of the experiment (brain electrical activity and questionnaires). Then it was time to figure out what we had.

The first thing we found was that anxiety symptoms fell about 12 percent among the people who took the MBSR class but increased slightly among the wait-list control group. The MBSR group also showed a significant shift toward greater left-side frontal activation: Compared with what it had been before the course, the level of left-side activation had tripled after four months. The control group actually had less left-side activation at the end of the study than they had at the start. (Maybe they were disappointed at not being in the MBSR group.) We also drew blood samples before and after giving everyone a flu shot, and here, too, we found effects of MBSR: Meditators produced 5 percent higher levels of antibodies to the vaccine, an indication that their immune systems responded more effectively than those of the control group. Intriguingly, participants who showed a larger brain response to MBSR also showed a larger response to the flu vaccine. That gave me confidence that brain activity and the immune system are indeed coupled, as I suggested in chapter 6: Positive emotions (being at the Fast to Recover end of the Resilience style and the Positive end of the Outlook style) boost the immune system, among other beneficial effects on bodily health.

MBSR can shift you toward the Fast to Recover end of the Resilience spectrum and the Positive end of the Outlook spectrum indirectly, by affecting your ability to deal with stress. That is, being better able to cope with stress means you are more able to bounce back from a setback, and it can cause you to see the world through more optimistic eyes. I suspect this works by retraining habits of mind. We all have habitual ways of responding to emotional challenges, and these habits are complicated products of genetics and experience. Mindfulness training alters these habits by making it more likely that one neuronal pathway rather than another will be used. If the habitual response to a setback had been for neuronal signals to travel from the frontal cortex, which figures out the meaning of an experience, to the limbic system, where the amygdala attaches an intense negative emotional valence to that experience, then mindfulness can create a different neuronal pathway. The same experience is still processed by the frontal cortex, but the signals do not reach the amygdala (or at least fewer of them do). Instead, they peter out, like a bad mood evaporating during a day when everything seems to go right. The result is that what had been a stressful experience or setback no longer triggers a feeling of anxiety, fear, or fatalistic capitulation. The habitual path traveled by neuronal signals has changed—much as water that had always followed one path along a stream can be diverted to a different course after a sudden storm, for instance, carving a new channel. Mindfulness meditation carves new channels in the streambeds of the mind.

More specifically, mindfulness trains the brain in new forms of responding to experience and thoughts. Whereas the thought of how much you need to accomplish tomorrow (driving children to school; going to an important meeting for work; getting a plumber to fix the leak under the sink; calling the IRS about the mistake they caught on your 1040; getting dinner on the table . . .) used to trigger a panicky sense of being overwhelmed, mindfulness sends thoughts through a new culvert: You still think about all you have to do, but when the sense of being overwhelmed kicks in, you regard that thought with dispassion. You think, *Well of course the sense of being overwhelmed is starting to course through my brain,* but you step back from it and let it go, realizing that allowing it to hijack your brain won't help. Mindfulness retrains these habits of mind by tapping into the plasticity of the brain's connections, creating new ones, strengthening some old ones, and weakening others.

That is why we found the brain changes we did. Our MBSR students showed greater activity in circuits in the left prefrontal cortex compared with the right, reflecting the fact that people practicing this form of mental training learn to redirect their thoughts and feelings (the physical manifestation of which is nothing but electrical impulses racing down the brain's neurons), reducing activity in the negative-emotion right prefrontal cortex and ramping it up in the resilience- and well-being-boosting left side. This new streambed carries more and more of your thoughts and feelings, creating a virtuous circle: The more your thoughts travel along the path of less anxiety, the greater your Resilience and the more Positive your Outlook, which makes it easier for thoughts and feelings to continue taking this new route.

Our Research Retreat

Other forms of meditation promise to affect one or more dimensions of Emotional Style even more directly than mindfulness-based stress reduction, as we were to learn in our next study. Most forms of meditation involve explicit instructions to regulate attention—to keep your focus on your breath, for instance. This often entails monitoring variations in attention, and if the mind begins to wander, gently bringing attention back to the breath. This made me wonder whether engaging in a form of meditation that cultivates attention causes attention to become more focused. Does it make you more aware of your surroundings? More self-aware? In other words, how do these practices affect any of the dimensions of Emotional Style?

To address some of these questions, we launched an unusual project in a setting very different from our usual research lab: a meditation retreat center in the quaint New England town of Barre, Massachusetts. There, in a wooded tract on the outskirts of town, the Insight Meditation Society (IMS) conducts intensive retreats in Buddhist-style meditation, mostly forms of mindfulness meditation that encourage practitioners to pay attention to the present moment in a nonjudgmental way. Most of the classes are held in the large main building, a former Catholic monastery with four imposing white columns in the front. Inscribed in the pediment above is the word *metta*, which is Sanskrit for "loving-kindness." In Buddhism, metta is the wish for all sentient beings to have happiness and its causes, and is one of the four "immeasurables" (the others are compassion, the wish that all sentient beings be free of suffering and its causes; sympathetic joy, the wish that all sentient beings never be separated from bliss without suffering; and equanimity, the wish that all sentient beings be free of bias, attachment, and anger).

In the summer of 2005, IMS graciously provided my research team with our own little house, where we set up a temporary laboratory in which we would test people before and after they undertook a three-month retreat. The retreat was quite intensive. Seven days a week participants woke up at five and spent the next sixteen hours—until bedtime, at nine—in complete silence, without making eye contact with anyone, even during meals. The only exceptions were during twice-a-week interviews with a meditation teacher, during which retreatants described their practice and any obstacles they were encountering. Retreatants spent their waking hours in meditation practice, eating, or doing an hour of daily work, typically cleaning or helping prepare meals, which were all vegetarian. Most logged more than twelve hours a day in meditation, or a thousand-plus hours over the three months. As you might imagine, it would have been too disruptive to test participants during the retreat, so we confined our work to the few days before they began and after they finished, three months later. For our control group, we enlisted people back in Madison, all age- and gender-matched to the retreatants.

We chose to study whether this intense meditation practice had any effect on attention—in particular, two aspects of it. The first is attentional blink, the phenomenon I described in chapter 3, which you almost have to see to believe. It refers to the fact that when information is rapidly changing in our environment and we are searching for particular stimuli, targets, or events, we are likely to be oblivious to those targets if they occur very close to one another, usually less than half a second apart. This might happen, for instance, in a computer game in which you have to capture certain kinds of creatures who pop onto the screen. If the second one follows the first by one-third of a second, you won't even see it (let alone be able to grab it with your mouse). It's as if after registering the first target, attention "blinks," thereby missing the second target.

Attentional blink is not just an arcane laboratory artifact; it occurs in the real world, too. We are constantly bombarded with a barrage of stimuli, even in relatively quiet environments. Think about the last time you had an important conversation. Many nonverbal gestures, subtle facial expressions, tiny eye movements, and the like form a key part of the conversation and convey important information. Yet these gestures and expressions occur so rapidly that attentional blinks cause you to miss a lot of them and thus fail to perceive signals that provide important social and emotional cues.

One hypothesis that psychologists have proposed to explain attentional blink is that the brain invests so much of its attentional resources in detecting the first target that there is not enough left to detect a second. Only after attention has "reset," or gotten its second wind, so to speak, can it perceive a subsequent target. A prediction of this "overinvestment hypothesis" is that if you can decrease the attentional resources needed to perceive the first target, you'll have enough left over to perceive the second, and thus your attention will not blink. This is why we thought meditation might be relevant: In vipassana meditation, you engage in what's called bare attention, which means directing your attention to present thoughts, emotions, and sensations but without judging those mental objects or becoming engrossed in them. We wondered if practice in bare attention might reduce the amount of attentional resources needed to detect an initial target, leaving more available to perceive a second one, thus eliminating attentional blink.

In our study, we presented a series of letters very rapidly, ten per second. Every once in a while, a number was inserted among these letters. The participants were asked to report each number they saw. So in a sequence like R, K, L, P, N, E, 3, T, U, S, 7, G, B, J (which would flash by in 1.4 seconds), people would have to notice the 3 and the 7. Most people have no trouble detecting the 3, but most of them miss the 7; their attention blinks. It is as if they get so excited that they detected the 3, their minds get fixed on that number and they are blind to the 7. We administered this test of attentional blink to all the retreatants before they began their intensive meditation, and then again after their three-month retreat, as well as to the control group. As expected, everyone was afflicted by attentional blink at the beginning, missing about 50 percent of the second numbers (though, as usual, there was individual variation). In addition to giving the performance test, we also measured people's brain activity using EEG. The visual cortex was, not surprisingly, quite active when people caught sight of the first number. But in people who missed the second target (which the soon-to-be meditators as well as the control group both did about half the time), this region was quiet.

Performance after intense meditation training was quite a different matter. The control group showed no improvement, which is what we expected. This ruled out the possibility that simply taking the attentional blink test a second time would improve performance. But the retreatants showed a marked decrease in attentional blink and thus a much greater ability to detect subsequent targets—on average, 33 percent more of the second targets.

The brain activity was even more intriguing. When someone did manage to perceive the second target, as more meditators did, her brain's attention region in response to the first target was not as active as it had been when she missed the second target. In other words, the amount of activation in the attention region in response to the first number predicted whether or not meditators detected the second number. Less activation in response to the first number was correlated with a higher rate of detecting the second number. This suggested that the overinvestment hypothesis was onto something: Attentional blink results from investing too much of our attentional resources in perceiving one target, leaving us too little to detect the second; but investing less in perceiving the first target leaves us enough to detect the second. Being able to focus attention in a calm, abiding manner without too much arousal or excitement maximized performance on this task—and that was the kind of attention participants had learned and developed after the three-month retreat.

We examined a second form of attention in the retreatants as well. Called selective attention, it reflects our capacity to tune in to certain stimuli and ignore others. People do this all the time, of course, since we could not possibly focus on all the stimuli that impinge upon our eyes, ears, and skin—for example, when you are driving you selectively focus (I hope) on the cars around you, not the feel of the seat belt across your chest. But what determines what we select? It might be the strength of the incoming signal: Perhaps the images of the cars produce stronger electrical activity in the brain than the feel of the seat belt. Or it might be signals that we mark as important: Perhaps some higher-order mental process does a quick scan of incoming information and boosts the strength of the car images but mutes that of the seat-belt feel. What we wanted to see was whether people can be intentionally selective rather than simply letting certain stimuli grab their attention because they are either stronger or more important.

To test this, we again invited soon-to-be retreatants to our little house at the IMS center. Once each person was comfortably seated and understood the protocol, we played tones through their headphones: a high-pitched tone and a low-pitched tone into each ear. As I described briefly in chapter 3, the participants were instructed to attend to only one type of stimulus in only one ear—for example, the high pitch in the right ear—and to press a button when they heard the target tone. After a few minutes of this, we changed the instruction, asking them to pay attention to only the low pitch in the right ear (and then the high pitch in the left ear, etc., until we had covered all four permutations). With tones arriving at a rate of about one per second, this wasn't easy, particularly when participants did it for twenty minutes at a stretch. On average, people missed 20 percent of the target tones, either failing to press the button when they heard the correct pitch in the correct ear, or mistakenly pressing the button when they heard the incorrect pitch in the correct ear or any pitch in the incorrect ear. (Needless to say, before administering the test we made sure a participant had normal hearing.)

Would three months of meditation practice that trains attention improve the performance on this task? After their retreat, we retested the meditators, as well as the control group. The latter had not improved, again showing that simple familiarity with the test didn't help. But the retreatants got significantly better: They responded correctly to more of the target tones and made fewer mistakes by pressing the button for tones they were supposed to ignore, getting it right 91 percent of the time, compared with 80 percent before their meditation training. Another finding was even more striking. The meditators, but not members of the control group, became much more stable in their performance. That is, the amount of time they took before correctly pressing the button was consistent, varying by an average of 110 milliseconds. In contrast, the controls as well as the retreatants themselves before their training sometimes responded slowly and sometimes quickly. (People with attention deficit/hyperactivity disorder are also inconsistent in their response time on this type of task.) After the meditation retreat, the variability in the participants' response time fell by 20 percent, whereas that of the control group actually increased.

Again, in addition to measuring performance, we recorded brain activity with EEG during this selective attention task. What jumped out at us was a measure called phase-locking. As you'll recall from chapter 4, this pattern of electrical activity reflects the degree to which brain waves—or, more formally, cortical oscillations—become synchronized to an external stimulus. With a high degree of phase-locking, an external stimulus triggers a clear pattern of cortical oscillations that are easy to pick out against the background oscillations—but only if the brain is not a jumble of mind-wandering and thoughts. In that case, the response to an external stimulus is as difficult to pick out against this background cacophony as the ripples from a rock splashing into a turbulent sea: There are so many other waves and disturbances that any ripples from the thrown rock are almost imperceptible. But if the rock lands in a perfectly still lake, the ripples stand out like a walrus in a desert. A calm brain is like a still lake. When an external stimulus comes in, it triggers clear oscillations synchronized to the arrival of the stimulus. The more a participant showed this phase-locking, the more accurate he was on the selective attention task.

An intriguing new study supports the finding that mental training can alter brain patterns that underlie attention. Scientists at the Massachusetts Institute of Technology and Harvard had half a group of participants practice mindfulness-based stress reduction for eight weeks, while the other half bided their time on a waiting list. Before the training began, the scientists took measurements similar to EEG, but rather than detecting electrical activity, they measured magnetic fields. Called magnetocencephalography (MEG), it uses an apparatus that looks like a giant hair dryer. MEG is more spatially precise than EEG, which came in handy: The participants were instructed to focus on their hand or their foot, a variation on the selective attention task I used at the retreat center. After the MBSR training, brain activity when participants focused on their foot changed in a very specific way: Alpha waves, which reflect cortical idling, increased in the part of the somatosensory cortex devoted to feeling the sense of touch on the skin of the *hand*. The control group showed no such increase. These findings add support to the idea that mindfulness meditation transforms the neural underpinnings of attention, in this case by minimizing activation in regions that are not relevant to the object of attention. Basically, the mental training helps the brain reduce background chatter and focus on selected information.

Can You Train Compassion?

With the discovery that even three months of meditation training can affect mental functions as basic as attentional blink and selective attention, I became more and more convinced that the brain changes that accompany meditation must occur pretty quickly. You don't have to wait until you are a meditation Olympian, with upwards of ten thousand hours of meditation under your robe. As it happens, this is the question I get most often when I talk about our studies of long-term practitioners: After people look at me askance, certain that they will not devote that much time to training their mind, someone always asks whether much shorter amounts of mental training can still be beneficial. I believe that with attention, the answer is yes, and in the next chapter I will describe a step-by-step program for producing the kind of changes we identified in the brains of the retreatants.

But what about some of the other qualities that are so striking in the monks? After the study at the meditation retreat, I was ready to try once again to study long-term meditators. I already had preliminary results from Matthieu Ricard. With his help, and the Dalai Lama's, I set out to see what else meditation might do to the brain.

The usual procedure in scientific research using human volunteers is to recruit as many people as you need up front and then run the study. That wasn't going to work with long-term meditators. You don't find many people who have done more than ten thousand hours of Buddhist meditation in one place, and certainly not in Madison. So we had to improvise. Soon after we had studied Matthieu's brain in conjunction with the Dalai Lama's visit, the word went out from the Dalai Lama and from Matthieu that if any adept meditator planned to be in the United States, and especially in the Midwest, to please get in touch with me before his trip so we might arrange a visit to my lab. To my delight, it worked. First I heard from Tenzin Rinpoche, a forty-one-year-old monk born in Tibet and living in India who was going to be teaching in the United States. Then I heard from Sopham Rinpoche, a fifty-four-year-old monk from Bhutan who agreed to fly to the United States just for this. Getting even the minimum number of subjects was a slow and painstaking process. But over the course of eighteen months I eventually got eight monks (including Matthieu), ranging in age from thirty-four to sixty-four, with ten thousand to fifty thousand hours of Tibetan Nyingmapa and Kagyupa meditation experience, to come to Madison and spend quality time with an EEG hairnet pasted to their scalps and meditate inside a claustrophobia-inducing tube that sounded like a jackhammer.

For the first study, I was interested in a phenomenon called neural synchrony. As you might infer from the name, neural synchrony means that individual neurons across widespread regions of the brain are firing at the same time. Research from other labs had linked the neural synchrony of high-frequency brain waves to mental processes such as attention, working memory, learning, and conscious perception; the suspicion is that by firing in sync, neurons cause far-flung networks to work together, with the result that cognitive and emotional processes become more integrated and coherent.

We followed the same procedure for each monk, so let me tell you about Tenzin Rinpoche. He came to the lab in the morning, and after explaining what we had in mind (much easier than with the monks in the hills above Dharamsala), we fitted him with a hairnet studded with 128 electrodes. The net keeps the electrodes mostly in place, but you still have to moisten each one to make sure the electrical contact is good—a laborious process that allowed ample time for discussing the experimental protocol and ensuring that he understood what would be required. My colleague Antoine Lutz, a French scientist who has been key to our studies with long term meditation practitioners, took the lead. First he asked Rinpoche to simply sit, keeping his mind neutral, for sixty seconds at a time. After several rounds of this to establish a baseline of electrical activity, we then switched to meditation. Antoine asked Rinpoche to begin "unconditional compassion" meditation. Matthieu, who helped design the study, describes the resulting meditative state as "unrestricted readiness and availability to help living beings." This form of meditation does not require concentrating on particular objects, memories, or images; it simply generates feelings of benevolence and compassion, causing them to "pervade the mind as a way of being." This state is called pure compassion or nonreferential compassion (*amigs med snying rje* in Tibetan). Twenty seconds later, we began EEG recording. We took data for sixty seconds and then asked Rinpoche to switch off the meditation. He rested for thirty seconds, then we repeated the sequence three times, for a total of four meditation blocks. We repeated the same procedure for Matthieu and the other six monks who eventually came to Madison. "We tried to generate a mental state in which compassion permeates the whole mind with no other consideration, reasoning, or discursive thoughts," Matthieu explained later.

For our control group, we recruited Madison undergraduates and gave them a crash course in compassion meditation. We asked them to think of someone they cared about, such as their parents or a significant other, and to let their mind be pervaded by feelings of love or compassion (in the latter case, by imagining the person in a sad or painful situation and wishing that he or she be free from suffering). After trying this for one hour, the controls attempted to generate that feeling not merely toward one person but toward "all sentient beings," without thinking specifically about any individual.

I didn't want to jump to conclusions based on the results of a single meditator, but as soon as I looked at the EEG data from Rinpoche, I suspected that something remarkable was going on. Once I had data on all eight, I was sure. For one thing, during meditation gamma activity was greater than had ever been reported in the scientific literature. Gamma waves are high-frequency brain waves that underlie higher mental activity such as consciousness. Although the control group that had just learned compassion meditation showed a slight increase in gamma activity, most of the monks showed extremely large increases. Since the size of the gamma wave is related to the number of neurons firing in sync, this was evidence for massive, far-flung assemblies of neurons firing with a high degree of temporal precision, like Rockettes kicking as one from one side of the vast Radio City Music Hall stage to the other. Gamma waves increased gradually as the meditation went on, which reflects the fact that neural synchronization requires time to develop. Since neural synchrony underlies many higher mental processes such as perception and attention, I took this as intriguing evidence that meditation might produce fundamental changes in brain function, which would have important implications for our ability to learn and perceive. In particular, high gamma-wave activity and neural synchrony might be the brain signature of what the Buddhist practitioners themselves report they experience during meditation: a change in the quality of moment-to-moment awareness, bringing with it a vast panorama of perceptual clarity. It is as if a mental fog lifts, one that you did not even realize had been impeding your perception.

Using fMRI, we pinpointed regions that were active during compassion meditation. In almost every case, the enhanced activity was greater in the monks' brains than in the control group's. Activity in the insula, a region important for the bodily signals associated with emotion, and in the temporoparietal junction, which is important for empathy, was dramatically amplified in the long-term practitioners. A sprawling circuit that switches on at the sight of suffering also showed greater activity in the monks. So did regions responsible for planned movement, as if the monks' brains were itching to go to the aid of those in distress. When I asked Matthieu what might explain this, he thought about how compassion meditation feels, especially when he thinks of a loved one in distress, and described it as "like a total readiness to act, to help."

Even more intriguing to me than the increase in neural synchrony during meditation were the EEG readings from when the monks were in their baseline state—resting quietly but not meditating. Here, too, gamma activity and neural synchrony were significantly greater than in the controls. This was a hint that meditation is not only marked by characteristic patterns of brain activity (which isn't that surprising, really), but that it produces enduring increases in gamma activity and neural synchrony. Maybe, I thought, the attention required for the meditation and the compassion it generates are skills that can be acquired or enhanced through training.

I couldn't rule out the possibility that there was a preexisting difference in brain function between monks and novices, and that these differences were the cause of the much greater gamma synchrony. But the fact that monks with the most hours of meditation showed the greatest gamma synchrony, both at baseline and as an increase during meditation, gave me confidence that the changes are actually produced by mental training—a hypothesis I raised in the 2004 paper describing this study.

Focus, Please, Rinpoche

Since monks willing to spend hours having their brains studied were not exactly in great supply, I risked wearing out my welcome by asking them to participate in another, parallel study. After they switched compassion and loving-kindness meditation on and off for us while wearing the EEG hairnet and then in the MRI tube, I prevailed upon them to do something similar with a form of meditation called one-pointed concentration. In this practice, the meditator focuses on a single object of attention, such as the breath or a picture or statue of the Buddha, strengthening the attentional focus until he achieves a tranquil state in which preoccupation with other thoughts and emotions is gradually eliminated; nothing but the focus on the breath or the Buddha fills the mind. At the same time, the meditator engages in self-monitoring, noting any thoughts or mental states other than the concentration on, for example, the breath. He may notice sleepiness, or he may make note of when "mental chatter" begins to intrude. Matthieu explains the concentration state as one in which "one tries to focus all one's attention on one object, keep it on that object, and bring it back to that object when one finds that one has been distracted by outer perceptions or inner thoughts. You resist sinking into dullness or sleepiness, or being carried away by mental agitation and internal thought chatter. If you experience this, calmly but deliberately return to the object of meditation with a sense of sharp focus." For the neutral state, the eyes remain open as they do during meditation, Matthieu explains, and "your emotional state is neither pleasant nor unpleasant. You remain relaxed. Try to be in the most ordinary state without being engaged into an active mental state, like voluntarily remembering or planning something or actively looking at an object."

Our study of the retreatants at the meditation center in Barre had already shown that an intense course of meditation could improve selective attention and decrease attentional blink. I wondered what upwards of ten thousand hours of meditation might have done.

In the study, we had to work within the confines of the MRI tube, so for the focus of concentration we decided to project a dot on a screen mounted on the ceiling of the tube. Once the monk settled in, Antoine Lutz asked him to turn his meditation on and off, according to a script that we had calibrated with the software. After ninety seconds of rest, Antoine asked the monk to switch on attention meditation ("Shamatha, please, Rinpoche"), which the monk would sustain for two minutes and forty seconds. Then Antoine said, "Lung ma bstan," and the monk would return to a neutral state for about ninety seconds, all repeated for a total of ten cycles. It took about eighteen months to gather data on a total of fourteen visiting monks, as well as twenty-seven controls (again, students who were given a one-hour crash course in concentration meditation and practiced it for a total of four to five hours in thirty-minute chunks before the experiment started).

The first thing we saw was exactly what we had expected: Brain networks that underlie vision and attention were more active during meditation than during resting. In particular, the dorsolateral prefrontal cortex (which monitors the environment for objects demanding attention), the visual cortex (seeing), the superior frontal sulcus, the supplementary motor area, and the intraparietal sulcus (all involved in attention) were much more active during meditation than during rest, in the monks as well as in the novice meditators. No surprise there. But the devil, or in this case the angel, was in the details. The novices had less activation in the attention regions than the expert meditators as a whole. But when we divided the experts into two groups, one with 10,000 to 24,000 hours of meditation experience and the other with 37,000 to 52,000 hours, we saw something more interesting: Although the monks with fewer hours of practice had more activation of the attention networks than the novices, the monks with the most hours had *less* activation. The graph looked like an inverted U: Activation rose and rose as the number of hours a meditator had practiced rose, but then fell as the number of hours of practice increased beyond 25,000 or so.

This reminded me of how a dedicated amateur cyclist will pump harder and faster than a bicycling novice while getting up a steep hill—reflecting greater muscle capacity—but a Tour de France–caliber cyclist will ascend the same hill almost effortlessly. The most experienced meditators were able to maintain their focus and concentration with even less effort than the controls. This matched what the monks told us. When they first practiced this form of meditation, it required significant effort, but as they became more accomplished they were able to attain a "settled state" of alert focus with minimal effort. This also describes what a monk experiences in a meditation session, when some effort is required to first reach the state of alert focus but then he settles into it, and less mental effort is required to maintain the same attentional focus. This also squared with what we found in the Barre retreatants when we gave them the attentional blink test: With meditation practice, their mental activity became quieter but no less effective, with the result that they were able to notice the first stimulus with only minimal attentional effort, reserving enough to notice the second.

How did we know the experts who showed so little activation in the attention circuit weren't actually letting their minds drift to thoughts of, say, getting the heck out of the noisy MRI tube and grabbing some lunch? Because during their concentration meditation, every six to ten seconds we piped two seconds of sound into their headphones (which are necessary so the participants can hear sounds over the loud pounding of the MRI tube), either something neutral such as ambient noise recorded in a bustling restaurant, something pleasant such as a baby cooing, or something disturbing such as a woman screaming. This would seem like enough to distract anyone, but that was not the case. Upon hearing any of the sounds the novices did indeed show a reduction in activity in their attention regions as they lost their focus on the dot. The medium-term meditators had some reduction in activity there as well. The novices also showed increased activity in brain regions associated with unrelated thoughts, daydreams, and emotional processing—the latter probably a reflection of their annoyance at having their concentration disrupted. The expert meditators showed no such increase in distraction-related regions. They maintained their focus. They also had less activation than the controls in the amygdala in response to the emotional sounds. Again, activation was correlated with hours of practice, with more hours leading to less activation. This finding supports the idea that advanced levels of concentration can keep emotional reactivity in check, especially when that reactivity can disturb concentration.

This study, which we published in 2007, provided strong evidence that the brain's attention systems can be trained. Like any form of workout, from weight lifting to cycling to learning a second language, it causes an enduring change in the system that is engaged. In this case, that change is the ability to maintain laser-sharp concentration with less and less activity in the brain's attention circuit.

Loving-Kindness in a (MRI) Tube

I wanted to learn more about the lasting effects of compassion and loving-kindness meditation, and again Matthieu was instrumental in making this a reality. This time he helped me recruit sixteen long-term meditators, and I advertised for people who might be interested in learning compassion meditation. To give you a sense of what this form of meditation involves, let me quote how Matthieu explained it to our recruits, who got a crash course from him (one hour of instruction plus another four hours of practicing on their own). "During the training session," Matthieu told them, "you will think about someone you care about, such as your parents, sibling, or beloved, and will let your mind be invaded by a feeling of altruistic love (wishing well-being) or of compassion (wishing freedom from suffering) toward them. After some training you will generate such feeling toward all beings and without thinking specifically about someone. While in the scanner, you will try to generate this state of loving-kindness and compassion until an unconditional feeling of loving-kindness and compassion pervades the whole mind as a way of being, with no other consideration or discursive thoughts." We used the same basic approach as we did in the study of attention meditation, asking the monks and the novices to alternate between resting states and meditation states while in the MRI.

Buddhist tradition teaches that as a result of compassion meditation feelings of empathy arise more readily, effortlessly, and often accompanied by a desire to act for the benefit of others. We weren't going to take our volunteers to the site of a highway crash and see how they behaved, but the brain activity we measured suggested that the tradition had gotten it right.

As in the attention study, we played sounds while the volunteers were in the MRI tube, either neutral ones (the restaurant), pleasant ones (the cooing baby), or distressing ones (the screaming woman). In monk after monk, the strength of the activation in response to the woman's screams was greater during compassion meditation than in the resting state—and greater than the response of the novice meditators. We saw this with spikes of activity in the insula, which is essential for activating bodily responses that play a role in feeling another person's suffering and thus in empathy. Activity in this region rose (although not as much as in response to the sound of the woman screaming) when our volunteers heard the cooing baby, too—again, more in the expert meditators than in the novices, and more in the meditative state than in the resting state—supporting the traditional Buddhist view that compassion meditation enhances the feeling of loving-kindness in response to the joy of others. In fact, when our monks and novices reported that a particular session of meditation was unusually successful in cultivating compassion, activity in these empathy regions was greatest of all.

There was also greater activation in the monks than in the novices in a circuit that has been linked to reading other people's emotional and mental states, including regions called the medial prefrontal cortex, the temporoparietal junction, the posterior superior temporal sulcus, and the posterior cingulate cortex. There was greater activity in the right than the left side of several of these regions, especially the temporoparietal junction and posterior superior temporal sulcus, a pattern that is associated with self-reported altruism. The greater increase in activation of this circuitry in experts than in novices suggests that experts might be more primed to detect the suffering of others.

The pattern of brain activity when people were *not* meditating was equally intriguing. As I have said before, a measurement like this hints at whether meditation causes enduring changes in the brain, changes that persist as a background condition even when one is not engaged in meditation. EEG measurements showed that gamma oscillations in the prefrontal cortex were much more pronounced in the brains of the expert meditators than in those of the novices, with a notable increase in activation in regions associated with attentiveness. Compassion meditation, it seems, resets the brain so that it is always prepared to respond to another's suffering. The response itself will differ depending upon the circumstances, but compassion meditation seems to change the brain—by enhancing gamma oscillations and by increasing activation in a circuit important for empathy—so that there is always *some* response. It is like having a paramedic team on standby: It is ready to go at a moment's notice, and so is a brain in which the capacity for compassion has been cultivated.

Speed Compassion

Having established that long-term meditation might produce changes in the brain that support greater compassion ("might" reflects the possibility I mentioned at the start of this chapter that a study like this cannot determine whether the monks' brains were like this as a result of meditation, or whether their unusual brains caused them to devote themselves to the contemplative life), I wanted to see whether short experience with meditation could do something similar.

In 2007, therefore, we recruited forty-one volunteers for a study that, we told them, would teach them a technique to improve well-being. We randomly assigned everyone to either a meditation group or a group that would learn something called cognitive reappraisal. Derived from cognitive therapy, cognitive reappraisal is a technique in which—to oversimplify—you take a belief that is having harmful effects and ask yourself whether it is really true. For instance, someone who is suffering from depression and believes that she has no skills or talents will learn to adopt the attitude that she does have certain terrific skills but that many people do not perform well in certain circumstances; it doesn't reflect poorly on her, she learns to tell herself, but may simply be a consequence of the situation. Moreover, the person would be encouraged not to avoid future situations like the one in which this feeling first arose; that way, she can experience feeling okay in that situation. In therapy, this is accomplished by pointing out errors in thinking that produced these beliefs; the therapist and patient work together to challenge these errors and to minimize subsequent avoidance of the problematic situation. This helps the person differentiate between internal causes and external causes; by attributing fault to the latter rather than the former, studies have shown, cognitive reappraisal can significantly improve well-being among those suffering from depression. Although the technique might sound somewhat simplistic, cognitive reappraisal is one of the most well-validated psychological treatments for depression and anxiety disorders.

The meditation group learned a form of compassion meditation. The basic idea is to visualize and contemplate different groups of people. You start by visualizing a loved one—specifically, a loved one at a time in her life when she was suffering. With this image clearly in mind, you next concentrate on the wish that her suffering end, silently repeating a phrase such as "May you be free from suffering; may you experience joy and ease" to help you focus on this task. You also try to notice any visceral sensations that arise during this contemplation, particularly around the heart—a slowing heartbeat, perhaps, or stronger beating, or warm sensations in the chest area. Finally, you also try to feel the compassion emotionally and not simply think about it cognitively. After doing this for a loved one, you expand your circle of compassion little by little, to yourself, then to someone you recognize but do not really know (the letter carrier, police officer, bus driver . . .), then perhaps a neighbor or a person who works in the same building as you but whose life you know little or nothing about, then to a difficult person (someone who pushes your buttons and makes you angry), and finally to all of humankind. Using an online instructional program, this group practiced compassion meditation thirty minutes a day for two weeks.

Participants in the cognitive reappraisal group also began by visualizing the suffering of someone they loved but were told to "reframe" the suffering. Reframing is a technique in which you adopt different beliefs about the causes of your behavior or of the circumstances of your life. In this case, you see that the suffering might not be as extreme as other forms of suffering and that it could end up okay, or you focus on the fact that there are huge differences in the magnitude and severity of adversity. They were further taught to not attribute negative things to stable qualities in themselves but to see that suffering can occur as a result of external circumstances. For instance, the reason

someone might be unable to find a life partner is not because of anything inherent in himself, but because his work keeps him from getting out and meeting people—the latter being something we can control and that can change.
The cognitive reappraisal group also received their instruction online, also for
thirty minutes a day for two weeks.

As usual, before the training began we performed brain scans of all the
participants. While a volunteer was lying in the MRI tube, we presented pictures of human suffering, such as a child who had been badly burned or a
family in a horrific car crash. We focused on the amygdala, which is known to
be involved in feelings of distress. Perhaps counterintuitively, we predicted
that after compassion training this region would not be as active in response
to images of suffering. The reason is that activity in the amygdala is associated
with distress. Feeling distress interferes with the desire to help—the hallmark
of compassion—because if you are in pain yourself, you have little reserve for
others' pain. In addition, we predicted that the prefrontal cortex would become
more activated because, as the site of higher-order cognitive functions, it holds
within its intricate circuitry the neuronal representation of the goals of compassion training—to alleviate suffering in others.

At the end of the two weeks of training, we again recorded brain activity
with fMRI while the volunteers looked at images of suffering. Those who had
undergone training in compassion meditation showed striking changes in
brain function, particularly in the amygdala: Participants in the compassion
group tended to show less activation there in response to images of suffering
after the compassion-meditation training than they did before the training.
Might this be a habituation effect, a lab version of the "compassion fatigue"
people feel when they see one human tragedy after another? Not according to
our control group: In people who underwent training in cognitive appraisal,
amygdala activity in response to images of suffering was just as high as before
their training.

This decrease in amygdala activation after compassion training had real-
world effects, too. After their two weeks of training, we had each participant
play an economic decision-making game that is designed to measure altruistic
behavior. To earn up to thirty dollars (a meaningful sum to students), they
were invited to play an online game with live opponents who were in a different building on campus. (In reality, there were no human opponents; they were

playing against a computer. We tried to convince them that there were humans on the other end of the Internet connection by pretending to phone a scientist who was supposedly with the opponents and who requested more time for them to read the instructions.) Once all the participants were ready, we explained that the game has three players: a dictator, a victim (let's call her Jo), and you. Everyone but Jo gets thirty dollars to start. The dictator gives Jo a certain amount of his money. If he gives her very little, perhaps five dollars, the participant can spend some of his own money to make the transaction fairer, perhaps ten dollars. Whatever the participant gives is also taken away from the dictator and given to Jo, who in this example gets twenty dollars plus the original five. The participant has his original thirty dollars minus ten.

The experimenter then left the room, giving the participant complete privacy to make his decision. This design ensured that the participant's decision was not due to implicit pressure that he might experience from having the experimenter look over at him as he made his decision. We analyzed the data only from the 75 percent of participants who believed this setup.

You might expect that someone who is not feeling much distress—as shown by low amygdala activity—in response to someone else's "suffering" (though, admittedly, Jo's suffering was at the low end of the scale) would not be moved to alleviate that suffering. But the opposite is the case. Participants who had undergone training in compassion meditation, and whose amygdala activity in response to images of suffering had decreased, were much more likely to give Jo some of their earnings. On average, they forked over 38 percent more money than those who had undergone cognitive reappraisal training.

From this, we concluded that compassion meditation produces a trio of changes. First, it decreases personal distress, as reflected in decreased activation of the amygdala. Second, it increases activation in regions of the brain associated with goal-directed behavior, as reflected in increased activation of the dorsolateral prefrontal cortex (the goal in this case is to relieve the suffering of the player who gets taken advantage of by another player). Third, it increases the connectivity between the prefrontal cortex, the insula (where representations of the body occur), and the nucleus accumbens (where motivation and reward are processed). Rather than becoming depressed by suffering, people who are trained in compassion meditation develop a strong disposition to alleviate suffering and to wish others to be happy.

*   *   *

Let me recap what our studies of long-term meditators as well as the effects of a relatively short course of meditation have shown:

• Mindfulness-based stress reduction enhances left prefrontal activation; this is a marker of the Fast to Recover end of the Resilience continuum and is associated with greater resilience following a stressful challenge.

• A more intensive period of mindfulness meditation improves selective attention and reduces the attentional blink, moving people toward the Focused end of the Attention continuum. In both cases, mindfulness strengthens prefrontal regulation of brain networks involved in attention, in part by strengthening the connections between the prefrontal cortex and other brain regions that are important for attention.

• Compassion meditation can nudge you toward the Positive end of the Outlook dimension; it strengthens connections between the prefrontal cortex and other brain regions important for empathy.

• Compassion meditation also likely facilitates Social Intuition.

• While you might expect most forms of meditation to nurture Self-Awareness, at least the kind that makes you more attuned to bodily sensations such as heartbeat, we found that neither Tibetan forms of mindfulness meditation nor Kundalini yoga forms of meditation were associated with better performance on a task that measures awareness of one's heartbeat.

• Finally, we know very little about whether different forms of meditation impact the Sensitivity to Context style; there is no systematic research on how well someone can modulate his emotional responses based on social context.

In the final chapter, I turn to specific techniques that might be used to change where you fall on each dimension of Emotional Style.

CHAPTER 11

∎ ∎ ∎

Rewired, or Neurally Inspired Exercises to Change Your Emotional Style

What you've read about the discovery of Emotional Style, its origins in childhood, and the discovery of the brain patterns that determine where we fall along each of the six dimensions reflects my own serendipitous scientific journey, one driven by the conviction that emotions deserve primacy of place in the study of the mind no less than thoughts do. Without setting out to do so, I found that each of us is a color-wheel combination of the Resilience, Outlook, Social Intuition, Self-Awareness, Context, and Attention dimensions of Emotional Style, a unique blend that describes how you perceive the world and react to it, how you engage with others, and how you navigate the obstacle course of life. My scientific journey has culminated in the studies on long-term meditators described in the previous chapter, showing that we have the power to live our lives and train our brains in ways that will shift where we fall on each of the six dimensions of Emotional Style. And that is what we turn to now.

Let me dispense quickly, albeit respectfully, with the "I'm okay, you're okay" school of thought. As I alluded to in chapter 1, there are some Emotional Styles, some set points along each of the six dimensions, that simply make life more difficult and painful than it probably needs to be. I am definitely not arguing that everyone should aim for the middle of each dimension. I have known many productive, creative, fascinating people who embraced their gloomy view of life (Negative Outlook), their hypersensitivity to Context, their lack of Resilience, and their acute Self-Awareness—people who could not imagine being who they are with even a slightly different Emotional Style. Even if that, or something like it, describes you, however, while you might want to retain the pessimistic, neurotic, sensitive qualities that make you *you*, perhaps you would like to tweak your Attention dimension, or some other aspect of your Emotional Style, if it is preventing you from forging the relationships and achieving the accomplishments you wish to.

Another reason to shift your set point is that some spots along each of the six dimensions will serve you better in particular situations. Maybe you find that a pessimistic, Negative Outlook spurs you to work extra hard (*This task has "disaster" written all over it, so I better give it my all and cancel my other commitments for the week*), but that moving closer to the Positive end of the Outlook dimension works better in social situations (*Okay, I know I can shine at this party; here I go*). In this case, being able to regulate your set point along each of these dimensions at will would allow you to respond to each situation in the most effective way you can.

This is possible, at least to some extent. You can vary how focused or broad your Attention is. You can adjust how quickly or slowly you recover from adversity. You can regulate your Outlook, seeing some glasses as half full and others as half empty. And you can train your brain to be more or less socially intuitive, self-aware, and sensitive to context. To be sure, there are limits to the range one can travel. Because we do not know how much plasticity the emotional brain is capable of, I cannot promise that you can move yourself from one extreme of, say, the Outlook dimension to the other, turning Cassandra into Pollyanna, but I believe you can shift several points (as counted in the questionnaires in chapter 3) in either direction. This is important because neither end of the continuum is necessarily better or worse than its opposite. Again, it depends on who you are, what you want, what works for you, what values you hold, and what your circumstances are. I know any number of scholars who firmly believe that to be content—to have, in the terminology of Emotional Style, a Positive Outlook—is to be clueless, dense, and oblivious. Or as someone I know puts it, "Anyone who's happy must not understand the situation."

Even if you do not go so far as to embrace the most Negative set point of the Outlook dimension, you need to be careful what you wish for. While most people will likely choose to move toward the Positive end of this dimension, strengthening their ability to sustain positive emotion, in fact an excessively Positive Outlook can be highly inappropriate and get us into trouble. People who have an extremely, unremittingly Positive Outlook are often unable to delay gratification. They have difficulty sizing up situations realistically, and their excessive optimism (*I might as well eat this hunk of cheesecake; I can just spend more time at the gym tomorrow;* or *I think I'll buy this great pair of shoes, even if they do bust my budget; maybe I can get some overtime this month*) causes them to make unwise decisions. As a result, they are unable to resist immediate temptations in order to achieve a more distant goal. For much the same reason, they may have difficulty learning from their mistakes: Their Positive Outlook causes them to see their error and its consequences as nothing to fret about, so they fail to absorb its lessons. (*Failed to get that job I interviewed for, apparently because I showed no enthusiasm? Oh well, I'm sure the next interviewer will overlook that.*) Recent findings suggest that some individuals with very high levels of positive emotion are also more inclined to engage in risky behaviors such as excessive alcohol consumption, binge eating, and drug abuse. They are also more likely to neglect threats, their blithe attitude blinding them to danger. An excessively Negative Outlook, in contrast, can sap motivation and wreck your social life as well as your work life. Assuming that nothing good will come of anything, you risk giving up on love, work, and life before you even try.

Similarly, it might seem at first glance that greater Self-Awareness is better than less. After all, who would not want to understand why they feel as they do and what their body is trying to tell them? But countless events occur inside our brains and bodies, most of which we are unaware of. That is not necessarily a bad thing. You don't want to be conscious of all the mental computations required to produce a grammatical sentence, for example; you would never utter anything again. Maybe you don't even want to be aware of all the bodily signals associated with emotion; if they are intense, such as spikes in blood pressure and heart rate, they might overwhelm you and interfere with your ability to think and see clearly. And you definitely don't want to be aware of the brain signals that regulate breathing and heart function; the information barrage would drown out everything else. A more realistic case of extreme

Self-Awareness is people who cringe at the very thought of wool or synthetic materials touching their skin, swearing it makes them feel as if insects are crawling on their bodies. Similarly, maybe you have a relative who insists she simply cannot eat (fill in the blank with someone's most annoying food phobia) since it makes her feel bloated or queasy or groggy. Rather than being neurotic behavior meant to call attention to itself, this hypersensitivity might reflect extreme Self-Awareness, a heightened ability to perceive sensations on the skin and in the digestive tract. There is a reason why nature built us so that we are oblivious to so much.

At this point, scientific evidence for the plasticity of some of the dimensions is stronger than for others. As a result, so is the strength of the evidence for what specific forms of mental training can shift your set point. More research is also needed to identify the optimal form of training for different individuals. But we are moving in the right direction, toward neurally inspired behavioral interventions—forms of mental training that, by targeting the patterns of brain activity and the specific neural circuits that underlie the six dimensions of Emotional Style, can change where you fall along the spectrum of each.

Although my work has focused on the brain bases of Emotional Style, shifting your set point for some or all the dimensions is not the only option. Rather than altering your Emotional Style so it better fits your world, you can change your world—your immediate environment and the way you structure your life—to better accommodate your Emotional Style. Take Mike, the autistic teenager I introduced you to in chapter 7. He minimizes how much he needs to interact with others, thereby reducing the toll that being around other people takes on his overreactive amygdala. Similarly, someone who is not particularly sensitive to social context and therefore has difficulty behaving appropriately in different situations might find a job in which he can work from home. That way he would not have to readjust his behavior and demeanor every time his social surround changed, such as from home to work and back again— something his hippocampus isn't very good at. And someone who falls toward the Slow to Recover end of the Resilience dimension might choose an occupation that rarely forces her to confront crises, thus protecting herself from the consequences of a sluggish prefrontal cortex. By being aware of your Emotional Style, you can craft a life that accommodates it.

But accommodation is not always possible; we don't necessarily get to choose to work from home, let alone make a major career switch. And even if you are able to change your physical or social surroundings, the benefits may be short-lived. The occupation you thought would spare you from having to constantly defuse crises, thus accommodating your lack of Resilience, does nothing to shield you from personal crises that there's simply no hiding from, whether the death of someone you love, a natural disaster, or illness. In contrast, changing your Emotional Style by tweaking the neural machinery that underlies it promises to be more enduring. In what follows, then, I will offer specific suggestions for how you can construct a world of work and relationships that plays to the strengths of your Emotional Style and accommodates its weaknesses, but I will focus on changing where you fall on each of the six dimensions by targeting their neural basis. It's the difference between reading large-print books and having laser eye surgery.

You might glance back at the questionnaires you filled out in chapter 3, to remind yourself of whether you fall at either extreme or in the middle for each of the six dimensions. That's your starting point. With that as a prelude, here are ways to alter your set point on each dimension of Emotional Style and to change your environment to better accommodate it.

Outlook

Deciding whether you would like to make your Outlook more Positive or more Negative involves more than taking stock of whether your current set point leaves you with low-grade (or worse) depression, at one extreme, or annoys friends and colleagues who can't stand your perpetual Panglossian view of the world, at the other. An excessively Positive Outlook, as described earlier, also impairs your ability to learn from mistakes and to postpone immediate gratification in favor of a greater payoff in the future. Indeed, the inability to delay gratification is a hallmark of an extremely Positive Outlook. Shifting your set point toward the Negative extreme will address both problems. An excessively Negative Outlook, on the other hand, can sap your motivation and suck the joy out of your relationships; becoming more Positive can add some sparkle to your perspective.

As you recall from chapter 4, a Positive Outlook reflects high activity in the ventral striatum (specifically, the nucleus accumbens, within the ventral striatum, which processes the sense of reward), the ventral pallidum (also interconnected with the ventral striatum, it is exquisitely sensitive to hedonic pleasure), and the prefrontal cortex, which through its planning function helps to sustain activity in the nucleus accumbens. A Negative Outlook reflects low activity in these regions and weaker connections between them. Judging from the popularity of books and Web sites that promise the secrets to greater happiness, I'm betting more people want to increase their ability to sustain positive emotion than to let the blues linger. That means raising activity in the ventral striatum or the prefrontal cortex, or both, and increasing the strength of the connections between them.

A chief function of the prefrontal cortex is planning. You can therefore strengthen it much as you would strengthen your biceps: Exercise it. When you find yourself in a situation in which you are tempted by an immediate reward but you know the smarter, safer, healthier, or otherwise better choice is to wait for a future reward of higher value, pause and focus on the more valuable future reward. This can be looking at the plate of brownies you baked for dessert and, rather than having just a little taste (ahem) at three o'clock, conjuring up a mental image of dinnertime. See yourself carrying in the brownies. Imagine feeling guilty that you are about to have your second. Envision your waistline, or your cholesterol level. Now imagine enjoying the brownie with your family or friends because you know you have not overindulged. If necessary, find a distraction to divert your attention from the three o'clock brownie. This strategy strengthens the planning function of the prefrontal cortex by requiring it to envision a positive future outcome.

What I'm about to suggest may sound as mad as telling an alcoholic to hang out at a bar, but here goes: Seek out situations in which an immediate reward beckons, and resist its lure. Don't make it too hard on yourself at first. If you want to resist the siren call of shopping, go someplace without your credit or debit cards, with only enough cash for an emergency. Then you can practice resisting what the store is pushing, and have an easier time of it knowing you can't make the impulse buy anyway. But by focusing on the benefits of using the money you save for, perhaps, your child's college fund or a down payment on a house, you will build up your resistance—strengthening your prefrontal cortex and ventral striatum—for when harder-to-resist promises of immediate gratification beckon. Practice this each day for about fifteen minutes, taking that long to visualize the future reward. Continuing with this example, once you have built up your ability to focus on the delayed reward, step it up by taking your credit card with you to the store. Don't berate yourself if you occasionally slip up; you're allowed to indulge occasionally. The point is that by exercising your capacity for forethought and planning, you strengthen your prefrontal cortex and its connection to the ventral striatum. Just be sure to reward yourself once tomorrow actually arrives: After you imagine putting off a self-indulgent purchase until you have paid for necessities, feel free to actually buy the item once that happens. That way, you train your brain to believe that your imagined future will eventually arrive.

Focus on different longer-term rewards on different days—health rewards, monetary rewards, relationship rewards. Try practicing this exercise daily for one week and see if it makes a difference. Although you won't be able to look inside your brain to see whether connections between the prefrontal cortex and the ventral striatum have been strengthened, if you find that you can more easily reevaluate the relative benefits of an immediate versus a longer-term reward and reject the former, then in all likelihood that's what has happened. And here's the payoff: a greater ability to sustain positive emotions.

Another way to strengthen connections between the prefrontal cortex and the ventral striatum is a technique called well-being therapy, developed by Giovanni Fava, of the University of Bologna in Italy. Designed to enhance the components of well-being—autonomy, environmental mastery, positive interpersonal relationships, personal growth, purpose in life, and self-acceptance— well-being therapy has been shown to move people toward the Positive end of the Outlook dimension, enabling them to sustain positive emotions. Although before-and-after brain scans have not been done, from everything we know about the brain circuitry underlying these components it's a good bet that well-being therapy strengthens the prefrontal cortex and its connections with the ventral striatum.

Every day for a week, do these three exercises:

1. Write down one positive characteristic of yourself and one positive characteristic of someone you regularly interact with.

Do this three times a day. Ideally, you'll write down a different trait each time, but if you're stuck on how "helpful" your office colleague is, that's okay.

2. Express gratitude regularly. Pay attention to times you say "thank you." When you do, look directly into the eyes of the person you are thanking and muster as much genuine gratitude as you can. Keep a journal; at the end of the day, note the specific times you felt a genuine, even if brief, connection with another person during the act of expressing gratitude.

3. Compliment others regularly. Keep an eye out for opportunities to do so, such as a job well done at work, a beautiful garden a neighbor created, or even a stranger's gorgeous coat. Look directly into the eyes of the person you are complimenting. In your journal, note the specific times you felt a genuine connection with someone you complimented.

After a week of this, spend a little time reflecting on what changes you noticed in your Outlook style. In all likelihood, you will find that positive emotions stick around a little longer and that your sense of optimism and possibility swells. (By the way, I don't recommend going around insulting people or being an ingrate if you need to throttle back your Positive Outlook. Instead, stick with the anticipation of possible future negative outcomes, as I describe next.) As with physical exercise, you'll probably need to find a practical maintenance routine. Once your Outlook has become as Positive or Negative as you wanted, it is important to sustain a level of exercise that is sufficient to maintain your set point in an optimal zone for you.

If instead of making your Outlook more Positive you would like to shift toward the Negative end of the dimension, then your goal is to lower activity in the nucleus accumbens or ventral striatum, or both, or weaken connections between them. If you feel that you are too Pollyannaish, carrying a Positive Outlook to unrealistic extremes, then you should envision potential negative outcomes. If considering an expensive purchase, spend time reflecting on the possible negative consequences of that choice. If you are tempted to buy a snazzy new car even though your current one runs fine, write down all the things that might go wrong with it or detract from its allure: the fact that its value drops by thousands of dollars as soon as you drive it off the dealer's lot; how much more careful you will feel you need to be while driving or parking so you do not get even a tiny scratch on it (something you stopped worrying about with your current car); how the monthly payments will force you to curtail spending on other things you enjoy.

If you need a quick fix, instead of or in addition to the exercises that will shift the neural underpinnings of your Outlook dimension, you can make changes to your environment to accommodate where you fall along this continuum. If you are trying to move toward the Positive end of the spectrum, fill your work space and home with upbeat, optimistic, gratifying reminders of happy times and people who give meaning to your life, such as pictures of people you love or places that you associate with a strong positive feeling. Change the pictures often, even once a week, so you do not habituate to them; you can keep the same people and places, just get different photographs of them. If you'd instead like to dial *down* your Positive Outlook, you might fill your home and work space with reminders of threats to your well-being, such as descriptions of natural disasters or news about environmental and economic threats. (Given the state of the world these days, that can be as simple as waking up to an all-news radio station or reading the morning's headlines.)

Much as Mike found an environmental accommodation that allowed him to function better in spite of his autism, so it is possible to alter your world so your Outlook style does not hold you back. The first step is finding like-minded people; there is no more uncomfortable feeling than to be the extreme Negative outlier in a group of glass-half-full types, or to be Little Miss (or Mr.) Sunshine among people whose default option is existential dread. In addition, since people toward the Negative end of the Outlook dimension often report low levels of energy, finding an occupation that is not too demanding and that does not extend beyond normal hours would be helpful; a Negative Outlook type in a deadline-fueled job such as finance or journalism is the sort of mismatch that brings misery. You might also find a good fit in an occupation that rewards seeing the worst in people or situations, such as security work, law enforcement, or creating angst-filled poetry.

Self-Awareness

"Blissfully unaware" is a misnomer: Being blind and deaf to what your body is trying to tell you is a good way to miss important signs of illness, whether a fever that signals an infection or a tightness in the chest that means a heart attack. Being Self-Opaque has consequences for relationships, as well: If you cannot tell that your blood pressure is rising and your heart rate is increasing because you are angry, then you do not have a chance to walk it off before you have a crucial meeting, attend a conference with your child's teacher, drive home during rush hour, or do anything else that anger can cause to go off the rails. On the other hand, being acutely Self-Aware is a road to hypochondria and panic attacks, as well as to paralysis in your emotional life: If you are constantly besieged by messages about your state of mind and heart (*Uh oh, I'm feeling nervous again;* or *Here comes that tidal wave of anger*), it can be tough to get on with life.

In chapter 4, I explained that individuals with high levels of Self-Awareness (emotional or physical) have greater activation in their insula, while those with little Self-Awareness have decreased activation. In the extreme, ultrahigh levels of insula activity seem to be associated with the hyperawareness of every little change in heart rate or respiration that sometimes occurs in panic disorder. To move yourself toward the Self-Aware end of this dimension, then, you need to increase insula activation; to dial it back, you need to decrease it.

Thanks to research on panic disorder, we know something about how to decrease the insula activity that makes us too Self-Aware. The best-validated treatment for panic disorder is cognitive-behavioral therapy. In this approach, patients learn to reframe or reappraise the significance of internal bodily cues. For example, if you experience chest pain or another sensation that you interpret as a danger signal, tell yourself you have many sensations that are perfectly innocuous, and in all likelihood this one is, too. This kind of cognitive reframing, by reducing insula activity, often reduces panic symptoms substantially.

An alternative to becoming less Self-Aware of your body, thoughts, and feelings by decreasing insula activity is to decrease the rest of the brain's reactivity to the insula's signals. Basically, the idea is to alter your relationship to your thoughts, emotions, and bodily sensations so that you do not become entangled in an endless, self-reinforcing loop (heart skips a beat; *I'm having a heart attack*; heart rate spikes; repeat) and leap to the conclusion that some aspect of what you are feeling portends doom. The trick is to keep your mind from ruminating in response to these internal cues. Rather than target the excessive Self-Awareness that comes from the insula, therefore, the idea is to reduce activity in the amygdala and the orbital frontal cortex, which form a circuit that assigns emotional value to thoughts and sensations. By reducing this circuit's activity, the brain can start perceiving thoughts, emotions, and sensations less judgmentally and less hysterically, so that we are not hijacked by our internal chatter. You're still very Self-Aware, but it's not debilitating.

One of the most effective ways to reduce activation in the amygdala and orbital frontal cortex is through mindfulness meditation. In this form of mental training, you practice observing your thoughts, feelings, and sensations moment by moment and nonjudgmentally, viewing them simply as what they are: thoughts, feelings, sensations; nothing more and nothing less. By learning to observe nonjudgmentally, you can break the chain of associations that typically arise from every thought. *Ugh, I have to stop worrying about work* becomes *Oh, how interesting that a thought about problems at work has entered my consciousness. Ouch, my knee is killing me* becomes *Aha, a signal from my knee has reached my brain.* If these observations start spinning off into judgmental thoughts, as they tend to (*I should have finished that project sooner than two minutes before the deadline!*), try to return to the process of mere observation.

Developing these mindful habits often takes considerable practice, though our research indicates that even short amounts of time can make a difference. Many people report benefits after just twenty minutes of practice.

The best mindfulness instruction I know of comes in a course in mindfulness-based stress reduction, the most widely taught form of secular mindfulness meditation in medical centers today. You can find courses by checking out the University of Massachusetts Center for Mindfulness Web site, at www.umassmed.edu/content.aspx?id=41252. Alternatively, you can get an instructional CD that provides detailed guided instruction in mindfulness meditation, such as those produced by Jon Kabat-Zinn or Sharon Salzberg.

If you want to give mindfulness meditation a try before taking a formal course, you can begin on your own with awareness of breathing:

1. Choose a time of day when you are the most awake and alert. Sit upright on the floor or a chair, keeping the spine straight and maintaining a relaxed but erect posture so you do not get drowsy.
2. Now focus on your breathing, on the sensations it triggers throughout your body. Notice how your abdomen moves with each inhalation and exhalation.
3. Focus on the tip of the nose, noticing the different sensations that arise with each breath.
4. When you notice that you have been distracted by unrelated thoughts or feelings that have arisen, simply return your focus to your breathing.

You can do this practice with your eyes open or closed, depending on which feels most comfortable. I recommend you try this for five to ten minutes at a sitting, ideally twice a day. As you feel more comfortable, you can increase the length of your practice sessions.

Once you feel that you've got the hang of mindful breathing, let go of your breath as the anchor of your attention and allow your focus to come to rest on the dominant content of your conscious mind at the moment—a thought, feeling, or bodily sensation. Cultivate awareness of what is occurring without thinking about it and without judging it.

You might also try something I practice, called the body scan:

1. Sit upright on the floor or a chair, keeping the spine straight and maintaining a relaxed but erect posture so you do not get drowsy.
2. Move your attention systematically around your body, from one location to the next—toe, foot, ankle, leg, knee. Notice the specific sensation at each, such as tingling or pressure or temperature. Don't think about those parts of the body, but experience the sensations. In this way you cultivate awareness of your body in the context of nonjudgmental awareness.

3. If you start to get lost in a chain of thought or feeling, you can reengage with your breathing to settle your mind.

I recommend trying the body scan for five to ten minutes, ideally twice a day. After a few weeks, you should find that your relationship to your inner thoughts, feelings, and sensations has changed: You are now able to experience them with less judgment, panic, or obsession. You can be aware of them without getting sucked into the vortex that they often create. By strengthening nonjudgmental awareness, you keep thoughts and feelings from hijacking your mind.

Paradoxically, one of the most effective strategies for increasing activity in the insula, and thus becoming *more* Self-Aware, is also to practice mindfulness meditation. A 2008 study found that people who have practiced mindfulness meditation every day for about eight years have a larger insula than people of the same sex and age who do not meditate. How can the same practice both increase and decrease Self-Awareness?

The answer lies in how Self-Awareness arises and what, exactly, we mean by it. If you are so overcome by internal sensations that you have trouble functioning, chances are you have normal levels of internal signals, thus likely normal levels of insula activity, but you react to these signals with catastrophizing thoughts and feelings. In this situation, mindfulness meditation will transform your reactivity to the signals by turning down the volume on your amygdala and orbital frontal cortex. But if you have trouble discriminating internal bodily cues, mindfulness meditation can amplify them by increasing the gain on the insula. Mindfulness meditation, in other words, has a regulating effect on the mind. If you lack Self-Awareness, it can help make internal sensations more salient and vivid. If you are hyperaware, feeling and hearing your internal signals all too vividly and loudly, it can bring about a kind of equanimity so you are not as bothered by this internal noise. That equanimity eventually helps the noise itself die down.

As with every dimension of Emotional Style, enduring change will come about through mental practice that shifts patterns of neural activity. But you can also rearrange your environment to encourage or discourage Self-Awareness. To boost Self-Awareness, decrease distractions and choose quiet environments, which make it easier to perceive internal feelings and sensations. They're the "signal" you want to perceive; the stuff around you is the noise. By decreasing the noise, you can increase the signal-to-noise ratio. To decrease Self-Awareness, do the opposite: Arrange things so you have more external stimuli to focus on. Keep a radio on, for instance, but don't let it become background noise. Multitask, checking e-mail while you watch TV or listening to music while you work. This will leave you with fewer attentional resources to devote to internal sensations, decreasing your signal-to-noise ratio.

Attention

A dead giveaway that you are too Focused is that your family or colleagues complain that you don't even hear them when you're working. Another clue: You focus so intently on one aspect of a situation that you miss the big picture, as in the student who attends so closely to the font, layout, and format of a term paper that she fails to notice that the essay itself is incoherent. Being Unfocused, on the other hand, is its own hell, one that a good part of the pharmaceutical industry is happy to address, especially if you are a school-age boy. You miss what people are telling you because you are off in your own world, you are often unable to finish one task before being distracted by another, and when you read you find that by the time you have reached the bottom of a screen or page, you have forgotten the stuff at the top.

The Focused extreme of the Attention dimension is the result of enhanced activation in brain regions, including the prefrontal cortex and the parietal cortex, that constitute a circuit for selective attention. The prefrontal cortex is critical for maintaining attention, while the parietal cortex acts as the brain's steering wheel, pointing attention to particular places and thereby focusing attention on a specific target. At the Unfocused extreme, in contrast, the prefrontal cortex is underactive and the attention is stimulus driven: Whatever occurs around you draws your attention. You veer from one stimulus to the next with no internal rudder to guide your attention. Improving focus therefore requires increasing activity in the prefrontal and parietal cortices.

If you are bothered by being too Focused, then your goal should be to reduce activity in the prefrontal cortex. This would open your mind to more input from the environment, including the child standing at the door of your home office and begging you to come play. This quality of attention is characterized by high levels of phase-locking to stimuli in your environment, in which those stimuli become synchronized to ongoing neural oscillations. The result is a more receptive attentional stance.

To improve focus, I again recommend mindfulness meditation. In recent research in my lab, we have found that long-term meditation practitioners, when engaged in the simple practice of focusing on an object, show higher levels of activation in the prefrontal cortex and parietal cortex. Follow the instructions in the Self-Awareness section for mindful breathing and body scanning. Once you feel comfortable with these practices, you can move on to focused-attention meditation, which is also known as one-pointed concentration:

1. In a quiet room free of distractions, sit with your eyes open. Find a small object such as a coin, a button on your shirt, or an eyelet on your shoe. It is important that the object of attention be visual, rather than your breath, your body image, or other mental objects.
2. Focus all your attention upon this one object. Keep your eyes trained on it.
3. If your attention wanders, calmly try to bring it back to that object.

Do this daily, initially for about ten minutes. If you find that you are able to maintain your focus for most of that time, increase your practice by about ten minutes per month, until you reach one hour.

If you feel that your attention is excessively focused and wish to broaden it in order to take in more of the world, then open-monitoring or open-presence meditation can nudge you toward that end of the Attention dimension. In open-monitoring meditation, your attention is not fixed on any particular object. Instead, you cultivate an awareness of awareness itself. I recommend beginning with a focused-attention meditation practice such as breath meditation, which will give you a basic level of attentional stability and make open-monitoring meditation easier. The basics are:

1. Sit in a quiet room on a comfortable chair, with your back straight but the rest of your body relaxed. Keep your eyes open or closed, whichever you find more comfortable. If your eyes are open, gaze downward and keep your eyes somewhat unfocused.

2. Maintain a clear awareness of and openness to your surroundings. Keep your mind calm and relaxed, not focused on anything specific, yet totally present, clear, vivid, and transparent.

3. Lightly attend to whatever object happens to rise to the top of your consciousness, but do not latch on to it. You want to observe the thinking process itself, perhaps saying to yourself, *Oh, I notice that the first thing I am thinking of as I sit down to meditate is . . .*

4. Give your full attention to the most salient current object of consciousness, focusing on it to the exclusion of everything else but without thinking about it. That is, you are simply aware of it, observing it as disinterestedly as possible, but do not explore it intellectually. Think of the object of attention as if it were an image in a frame in a museum, or in a movie, with no strong relevance to you.

5. Generate a state of total openness, in which the mind is as vast as the sky, able to welcome and absorb any stray thought, feeling, or sensation like a new star that begins shining. When thoughts arise, simply let them pass through your mind without leaving any trace in it. When you perceive noises, images, tastes, or other sensations, let them be as they are, without engaging with them or rejecting them. Tell yourself that they can't affect the serene equanimity of your mind.

6. If you notice your mind moving toward another thought or feeling, let it do so, allowing the newcomer to slip into consciousness. Unlike in Attention-strengthening forms of meditation, you do not try to shoo away the "intruding" thought, but allow your mind to turn to it. The key difference from the breath-focused meditation described previously is that in open-monitoring meditation there is no single focus to which the

attention is redirected if it wanders. Rather, you simply become aware of whatever is in the center of attention at any moment.

7. Turn to this new object of attention as you did the first.

8. Do this for five to ten minutes.

Many practitioners of this form of meditation find they develop a kind of panoramic awareness, in which they are cognizant of their thoughts and feelings as well as their external surroundings. A study we did in 2009 suggests why. Using EEG, we discovered that when people practice open-monitoring meditation it modulates their brain waves in a way that makes them more receptive to outside stimuli—that is, they experience phase-locking, a signature of Focused Attention. Recall the lake metaphor in the previous chapter: If you toss a rock into a still lake, you can see the ripples very clearly; but if the lake is turbulent, you'll have trouble making out the change produced by the rock. In the same way, if our minds are still, we will be receptive to incoming stimuli, which is expressed as the phase-locking of cortical oscillations to these stimuli.

A number of meditation centers offer courses in open-monitoring meditation, including the Insight Meditation Society, in Barre, Massachusetts; Spirit Rock Meditation Center, in Woodacre, California; and Tergar, in Minneapolis. You can also find instructions online and in CDs and books from these centers. Transforming your skill in attention will require some practice, but because attention is the building block for so much else, I believe it's worth the effort. And I'm confident that most people will experience some benefit in a short period of time.

As with the other dimensions, you can arrange your environment to accommodate your Attention style, minimizing the chance that it will get in the way of what you want to achieve. To enhance your focus you need to minimize distractions. Clear out your environment, especially your work environment, eliminating as many extraneous stimuli as you can. That means as little noise as possible, especially conversations; if you can close your door, do so. Practice doing one thing at a time. If you are posting on Facebook or other social media sites, do that and that alone, without listening to music at the same time. When you use a computer, have only one program open: an Internet browser or e-mail program, but not both. If you are writing or using a spreadsheet or other

program, close your browser and e-mail, and disable any sound alerts for incoming messages.

If you are hyperfocused, you can try to create an environment to help you
broaden your attention. Scatter books and magazines around, tempting yourself to pick one up even if you are supposedly focusing on something else. If
you are working on the computer, keep the door to your room or office open so
you can hear the outside world, and have music playing in the background. If
you have a window, don't block it with curtains or shades, and try to position
your desk so you can easily glance up and look outside, where there are probably distractions galore. Place photos of loved ones near your desk so you can
glance at them as you work. Set the alarm on your cell phone or computer so
it chirps every twenty to thirty minutes and breaks your concentration, forcing you to take in the world around you.

Resilience

It may at first seem odd that anyone would want to be *slower* to recover from
adversity, but it is definitely possible to be too Fast to Recover. In order to have
a healthy emotional life, you need to be able to feel and respond to your own
emotions, which is difficult to do if you move on too quickly. Since we tend to
use the duration of an emotion as a marker of its intensity, being able to move
on after a setback may cause you to feel that your affect is blunted and that
you cannot experience emotions as intensely as you would like. In order to
have healthy relationships, you need to be able to feel and respond to other
people's emotions, meaning if you are extremely Resilient, others may perceive
you as unfeeling and emotionally walled off. Being very Fast to Recover, such
as after we witness someone else's pain or misfortune, can impair our ability
to experience empathy. Part of an empathic response is feeling someone's pain.
Indeed, recent research has shown that when we empathize, the brain activates many of the same networks as when we ourselves experience pain,
physical or otherwise.

It is easier to understand how someone might benefit from being faster to
recover. If setbacks leave you unable to function for long periods of time, it can
prevent you from achieving what you want and can make relationships diffi-

cult. Trapped in your own emotional morass, you may neglect family, friends, and work.

The brain signature of being Slow to Recover from setbacks is fewer or weaker signals traveling from the prefrontal cortex to the amygdala, as a result of either low activity in the prefrontal cortex itself or too few or less-functional connections between the prefrontal and the amygdala. Patients with depression who are Slow to Recover—every disappointment and setback shatters them—have very weak connectivity there.

Being Fast to Recover from adversity is a result of strong activation of the left prefrontal cortex in response to setbacks and strong connectivity between it and the amygdala. If you feel you need to boost your Resilience, you therefore need to increase activity in the prefrontal cortex (especially on the left side) or strengthen the neuronal highways between it and the amygdala, or both. If you feel you are so Resilient that you have cut off part of your natural emotional response to people, then your goal is to quiet activity in the prefrontal cortex and weaken its connections to the amygdala.

To cultivate greater Resilience and faster recovery from setbacks, I recommend mindfulness meditation. Because it produces emotional balance, mindfulness helps you recover, but not too quickly (just as it helps you focus but not get hyperfocused). Mindfulness weakens the chain of associations that keep us obsessing about and even wallowing in a setback. For instance, losing a job might cause your thoughts to tumble from "unemployment" to "no health insurance" to "lose home" to "I can't go on." Mindfulness strengthens connections between the prefrontal cortex and the amygdala, promoting an equanimity that will help keep you from spiraling down this way. As soon as your thoughts begin to leap from one catastrophe to the next in this chain of woe, you have the mental wherewithal to pause, observe how easily the mind does this, note that it is an interesting mental process, and resist getting drawn into the abyss. I recommend that you start with a simple form of mindfulness meditation such as the mindfulness of breathing, described previously.

If mindfulness practice does not move you as close to the Fast to Recover end of the Resilience dimension as you would like, cognitive reappraisal training can help. This technique, a form of cognitive therapy, teaches people to reframe adversity in such a way as to believe that it is not as extreme or enduring as it could be. For example, if you made a mistake at work and were barraged by distressing thoughts about it, you might think that you are not very smart, that you are likely to make the same kind of mistake again, and that the mistake is career ending. These errors in thinking are what cognitive reappraisal aims to correct. Rather than viewing the mistake as representative of your work, you are trained to realize that it was an anomaly and could have happened to anyone. Instead of thinking the mistake reflects something consistent and fundamental about you, you consider the possibility that you made the mistake because you were having a bad day, or didn't get enough sleep the night before, or because everyone is fallible. By challenging the accuracy of your thoughts, cognitive reappraisal can help you reframe the causes of your behavior and thus distress. This type of cognitive training directly engages the prefrontal cortex, resulting in increased prefrontal inhibition of the amygdala, the pattern that exemplifies resilience.

Cognitive reappraisal training is best conducted with a skilled cognitive therapist. The Beck Institute for Cognitive Therapy and Research, in Bala Cynwyd, Pennsylvania, which was founded by the inventor of cognitive therapy, Aaron T. Beck, has many online resources, including how to find a cognitive therapist in your community (www.beckinstitute.org).

If you instead wish to move toward the Slow to Recover end of the Resilience dimension, perhaps to strengthen your capacity for empathy, then you need to weaken connections between the prefrontal cortex and the amygdala. There is very little research on how to do this, but one strategy is to focus intently on whatever negative emotion or pain you are feeling as a result of a setback. This can help sustain the emotion, at least for a time, and increase activation of your amygdala. You can also focus on the pain of someone who is suffering, perhaps describing it in writing: *Nothing goes right for Aaron. His ex-girlfriend is using his credit card, his security job is in jeopardy because he got caught in an Internet sting, and his landlord is threatening eviction. He can barely get through the day anymore, and when he thinks no one is looking he cries and cries.* Use these descriptions to focus on the particular aspects of pain or suffering that you might feel in response. This exercise is likely to result in more sustained activation of the anterior cingulate cortex, insula, and amygdala, circuitry that is involved in pain and distress.

You can also engage in a type of meditation from the Tibetan Buddhist tradition called *tonglen*, which means "taking and receiving." Designed to cultivate compassion, it involves visualizing another person who might be suffering, taking in her suffering, and transforming it into compassion, and it is very effective at increasing empathy. To get started, try this exercise for five to ten minutes, four or five times a week:

1. Visualize as vividly as you can someone who is suffering. It can be a friend or relative who is ill, a colleague who is struggling at work, a neighbor whose marriage is ending. The closer the person is to you, the stronger and clearer the visualization will be. (If you are so fortunate as not to know someone who is suffering, try to visualize a generic person, such as a garbage picker in Delhi, a starving child in Sudan, a cancer patient in a hospice.)

2. On each inhalation, imagine that you take in this person's suffering. Feel it viscerally: As you breathe in, imagine her pain and anguish passing through your nostrils, up your nose, and down into your lungs. If it is too difficult to imagine physically taking in her suffering, then imagine the suffering leaving her each time you inhale. As you breathe in, conjure an image of pain and anguish leaving her body like fog dissipating under a bright sun.

3. On each exhalation, imagine that her suffering is transformed into compassion. Direct this compassion toward her: As you exhale, imagine the breath flowing toward her, a gift of empathy and love that will envelop and enter her, assuaging her pain.

There are ways of arranging our environments to accommodate variations in the Resilience style. To speed up your recovery from adversity, try to leave the situation where the setback occurred, if possible, and go to one with less emotional resonance. For instance, if you just had a fight with your spouse, leave the combat zone and walk outside, or at least into another room. To slow down your recovery and enable you to feel distress longer and more intensely, try do the opposite—remain in the situation associated with adversity or place reminders of it around you. For example, some people report that they feel no empathy for victims of natural disasters. If you want to become less unfeeling, try placing photographs of earthquake and tsunami victims on your refrigerator, for instance. That might help you feel their pain.

Social Intuition

It would seem as if everyone would want to shift their Social Intuition set point as close as possible to the Socially Intuitive end of the spectrum. After all, research on emotional and social intelligence argues that greater skill in these areas presages better success in love, work, and life in general. But it is also possible to be so focused on social cues and social events that they interfere with activities of daily living. If you cannot interact with coworkers without picking up the silent messages being transmitted between bitter competitors, for instance, you might very well have trouble functioning at your undistracted best.

The brain of someone who falls at the Puzzled end of the Social Intuition dimension is characterized by low activity in the fusiform gyrus plus high activity in the amygdala. At the opposite extreme, being Socially Intuitive reflects high levels of fusiform activation and low to moderate amygdala activity, giving you the ability to pick up even subtle social signals. While improving Social Intuition requires pumping up fusiform activity and quieting amygdala activity, reducing hyperintuition requires dialing down fusiform activity and ramping up that in your amygdala.

To increase fusiform activity in order to improve Social Intuition, the first step is to pay attention. To detect social cues, particularly subtle ones, you need to focus on what is going on around you: tone of voice, body language, facial expression. This is basically a matter of practice:

1. Start with strangers. When you are out in public, pick a couple or a small group of friends and discreetly watch them. Pay particular attention to their faces, which communicate so much social information. Remind yourself to look at other people's faces when you watch them and, particularly, when you interact with them.

2.　See if you can predict how they will touch each other (or not), how close they will walk together, whether they will look into each other's eyes while speaking.

3.　Get close enough to overhear them (assuming you can manage this unobtrusively; I recommend giving it a try in a crowded public place such as a party, a packed department store, or a jammed movie-theater lobby). See if their tone of voice seems to match their body language and facial expression.

4.　If not, then you are probably misunderstanding something. Take note of that, and apply this lesson to the next people you observe.

5.　Once you feel confident that you are able to tell what people are feeling, try it with friends or colleagues.

You can also cultivate Social Intuition through the mindfulness meditation described earlier. In this case, you can make the observation of social signals the objects of your mindfulness.

Now practice paying attention to people's eyes, which provide the truest signals about emotional state. At www.paulekman.com, Paul Ekman offers online training in micro-expressions, the fleeting facial expressions that punctuate social interaction. Because they are so brief, we often miss them and thus are oblivious to important social signals. Although research on whether such training can make you better at picking up social signals is still young, it's likely that any training to detect social signals increases activation in the fusiform area as well as the temporal sulcus, a region in the temporal lobes that is often activated in response to social stimuli. By making you more adept at reading the language of faces and eyes, this training should also cause you to fixate more on them, if only because they are now more meaningful and interesting to you.

Voice, posture, and body language also convey social and emotional cues. Specific exercises can increase your sensitivity to these other channels of communication:

1.　To enhance your sensitivity to vocal cues of emotion, when you are in a public place such as a subway, a busy coffee shop, a store where friends are chattering away, or an airport terminal, close your eyes and pay attention to the voices around you. Tune in to specific voices; focus not on the content but on the tone of voice.

2. Describe to yourself what that tone conveys—serenity, joy, anticipation, anxiety, stress, whatever. Test yourself by opening your eyes and observing what comes next. An encounter that ends with one party stalking away was more likely characterized by negative emotions than positive ones.

3. Now try that with posture and body language. As you observe a conversation, note how the speakers orient themselves toward one another, how they sit or stand, what gestures they make.

4. Designate one channel—tone of voice, body language—to be your focus of attention for a full day. As you commute, work, and observe family or friends or colleagues, look for opportunities to remove yourself a bit from the situation, even if only for a minute, so that you can be an observer and not a participant. Practice either steps 1 and 2, or 3, depending on which channel you are focusing on.

5. The following day, switch to the other channel and repeat the exercise.

I think you will be amazed at how this simple exercise can enhance your sensitivity to social cues in a short period of time.

If you feel so overwhelmed by the signals people transmit that you want to move closer to the Puzzled end of the Social Intuition spectrum, then you need to give your fusiform area a respite. (Just to be clear, this is specifically about receiving and perceiving fewer social signals, not reducing their effect on you; the latter is a function of the Resilience dimension, so if you feel that you are too much of a psychological sponge—absorbing the feelings of everyone around you, to your detriment—then use the exercises that move you toward the Fast to Recover end of the Resilience dimension.) Avoid looking at people's eyes. Use your Attention training to pull your focus back from intense concentration on people's body language and tone of voice. By engaging your fusiform area less, you will decrease its baseline activity and make yourself less intensely aware of the language of social signals.

There are a few ways you might alter your environment to accommodate your degree of Social Intuition. If you are at the Puzzled end of the dimension and content to stay there, arrange your routine so you spend relatively little time with people, particularly strangers. That will limit the situations in which you misread or are puzzled by social signals. Working from home can achieve the same thing. If, on the other hand, you are at the high end of Social Intuition and easily distracted by social cues, limit your social interactions to specific times of the day when they cannot knock you for a loop. Interacting with people during scheduled work breaks and meals, rather than off and on throughout the day, can limit this kind of disruption. If you are a student, studying in private rather than in a library, coffee shop, or other public place will keep social intrusions at bay.

Sensitivity to Context

Failing to correctly discern social context can lead to emotional responses that are appropriate in one setting but not another. It's appropriate to feel extreme anxiety in dangerous situations but not in safe ones; if you can't tell the difference, you are at risk for post-traumatic stress disorder. At the other extreme, which is less common, being too Tuned In to context can cause you to lose track of your genuine self: You may find that you alter your behavior to fit each different context. In this case, being a little more Tuned Out might be desirable. People who are very Tuned In to context tend to have strong connections from the hippocampus to areas in the prefrontal cortex that control executive functions and that hold long-term memories in the neocortex. People who are Tuned Out tend to have weaker connections.

There has been little research on how to strengthen or weaken these connections. The best clues come from research on PTSD, in particular the treatment called exposure therapy. This intervention consists of progressively more direct exposure to specific cues that are associated with the trauma, but in a safe context. For instance, if a woman has been assaulted on a dark city street and feels terror every time she leaves her apartment, the therapist might first teach her a breathing exercise that she can use to stay calm in the face of anxiety-producing cues. Then he might have her imagine the street where she was assaulted. Once she can manage that, the therapist might take her to the neighborhood that includes the street, and then to the street itself—always with someone she trusts and in broad daylight. Assuming the neighborhood is safe during daytime, this therapy would help the victim distinguish between the context of daylight and night. The essence of exposure therapy is to help patients implicitly process the safety of the current context in contrast to the danger of the traumatic context.

Based on the success of exposure therapy, we can surmise that a general strategy to enhance Sensitivity to Context is to gradually inure yourself to cues that make you anxious or angry:

1. To help you relax, start with a simple breathing technique from hatha yoga. With your eyes closed, attend to your breathing as you would in mindfulness meditation, counting the duration of each inhalation and exhalation.

2. Once you have counted for several breaths, lengthen your breathing cycle so it takes you one more second. Keep increasing the length as long as you feel comfortable, then maintain these longer breaths for five minutes.

3. Notice if the inhalation and exhalation are the same length. If one is longer, try to lengthen the other so that they take equal amounts of time. Do this for five minutes and then open your eyes.

Once you feel comfortable with this breathing exercise, move on to the context training. I'll use the example of a boss who makes you so anxious that you start sweating just thinking about him, with this anxiety spilling over into your family life. The same principle would work with any source of anxiety or dread:

1. Make a list of the specific cues and behaviors of your boss that upset you. Maybe he looms over your desk during the workday.

Maybe she loiters outside your work space at 4:55, watching to see if you leave even a minute early. Maybe he excoriates the reports or other work you hand in. Be as specific and vivid and detailed as possible.

2. Then, in a safe context such as at home on a weekend, gently and gradually bring to mind images associated with your boss. Conjure up exactly how she looks watching you at day's end. Imagine his face as he reads your work.

3. Simultaneously, perform the breathing exercise. Continue to do this until you feel comfortable and relaxed despite imagining your boss's glowering visage and his habit of hovering over your desk. Spend about fifteen minutes on this exercise.

You can expect to experience some benefit after doing this for four sessions, and the hour you invest will be well worth it. By improving your ability to distinguish between the context of your work and home, this exercise should help you distinguish among other contexts, too, and thus display context-appropriate emotional responses. Although there have not been any studies comparing brain activity before and after such training, the fact that exposure therapy helps PTSD patients suggests that it works by strengthening connections from the hippocampus to the prefrontal cortex and other areas of the neocortex.

There has been no research explicitly focused on moving people to the Tuned Out end of the Sensitivity to Context continuum, or on ways to weaken connections from the hippocampus to the prefrontal cortex and neocortex. But if you feel that shifting your set point away from the Tuned In extreme would help you stop tailoring your behavior to each context in a way that feels excessively contrived, I recommend the exercises that cultivate Self-Awareness. Becoming more mindful of your thoughts, feelings, and bodily sensations can help regulate your emotional responses so that they are not so easily affected by external context.

You can also arrange your environment to accommodate your Sensitivity to Context. If you are not very Tuned In, minimize the number of different contexts you find yourself in. Go to gatherings where there will be plenty of people you know, not a roomful of strangers. If you travel, try to do so with someone close to you; that way, although the physical surround will be new to you, the social one will be familiar and comfortable. If, on the other hand, you feel that you are so Tuned In that you feel compelled to adjust your behavior with every little shift of context to the point where you feel disingenuous, try limiting the range of contexts you inhabit in order to minimize the shifts in self-presentation that new situations trigger. This will remind you of core habits of mind that are consistent across contexts.

Changing Your Brain by Transforming Your Mind

All the exercises in this chapter work through the mind to change your brain. Whether inspired by millennia-old contemplative traditions or twenty-first-century psychiatric techniques, they have the power to alter the neural systems that underlie each of the six dimensions of Emotional Style. Any decision to shift your set point on any of these dimensions should be based on thoughtful introspection about whether it is keeping you from being the person you wish to be and living the life you aspire to. This, of course, requires awareness, something that, when it comes to understanding how we respond to emotional challenges, is in short supply. I hope the questionnaires in chapter 3 helped with that. I hope, too, that with this awareness you have seen that who you are today does not need to be who you are tomorrow, but that our Emotional Style is ours for the creating. Emotions help us appreciate others and the world around us; they make life meaningful and fulfilling. May each and every one of you flourish in your well-being and help others to do the same.

ACKNOWLEDGMENTS

There is not a day that passes without my deep reflection on and experience of gratitude for the extraordinary group of people I have had the privilege of working with in my laboratory and collaboratively over the years. This book is the culmination of thirty-five years of research work. In my graduate school days at Harvard, three of my mentors, Gary Schwartz, Jerome Kagan, and David McClelland, played a key role in teaching me about psychology as it was understood in those days and inspiring me to do what I do now; I owe much to them. What I learned then has provided a solid foundation for my more recent work, but much of what I do today as a practicing scientist—both the methods that I use and the concepts that guide me—were simply not available when I was a student. My work is really the product of a dedicated army of young graduate students, postdocs, and scientists, for whom I am so deeply grateful. An exhaustive list of former students and postdocs and collaborators would occupy many pages.

There is also a recency effect that has been described in psychology, in which we privilege information that has occurred most recently even though it may not be the most important. At the risk of committing this fallacy, however, I will name a few of the indispensable members of my lab, leaders of the key research projects that I have described in the previous pages. The studies of long-term meditation practitioners that are described in chapters 9 and 10 could never have been completed without Antoine Lutz. Antoine was the last graduate student of Francisco Varela, a great neurobiologist and one of the founders of neurophenomenology, as well as an early advocate of contemplative neuroscience, even though it was not named in Francisco's day. Francisco died prematurely of liver cancer in 2001. Antoine has been in my lab since 2002 and has been the key member of my team for our work with long-term meditation practitioners.

Our research on the neural bases of meditation, emotion regulation, Emotional Styles, and psychopathology has been carried out by an amazingly talented group of graduate students and young scientists whom I have had the privilege of working with over the years. They have included Melissa Rosenkranz, Helen Weng, Heleen Slagter, Kim Dalton, Brendon Nacewicz, Andy Tomarken, Daren Jackson, Carien van Reekum, Tom Johnstone, Heather Urry, Chris Larson, Jack Nitshcke, Tim Salomons, Jeff Maxwell, Alex Shackman, Aaron Heller, Drew Fox, Stacey Schaefer, Regina Lapate, Brianna Schuyler, Jamie Hanson, Sharee Light, Jessica Kirkland, Allison Jahn, and a crop of more recent students including David Perlman, Daniel Levenson, Joe Wielgosz, and Jenny Liu. Our translational research studies in our new Center for Investigating Healthy Minds has been made possible by two wonderful new scientists, Lisa Flook and Emma Seppela, and by our own in-house meditation teacher for our research with children, Laura Pinger.

In addition to these young scientists, I have been blessed with some extraordinary collaborators both here in Madison and throughout the world. Of special note was an early collaboration with Paul Ekman, one of the great psychologists of emotion. Paul took an interest in me and my career when I was just out of graduate school, and we have continued to interact ever since. The series of studies we did in the 1990s helped to lay the foundation for affective neuroscience.

Here at the University of Wisconsin my longest-standing collaboration is with my wonderful friend and colleague Ned Kalin. Ned is a talented psychiatrist and a very creative scientist. I have learned so much from him. Carol Ryff is the director of the Institute on Aging; I've collaborated with her on studies of aging and well-being. She has been an articulate voice of the importance of bringing the cultural and psychosocial worlds together with biology. Bill Busse, in the Department of Medicine, is one of the world's experts in asthma;

we would never have begun to study asthma without his direct involvement. Marilyn Essex, of the Department of Psychiatry, has been a wonderful collaborator on our studies of adolescence. She has tenaciously gathered an amazing dataset from a cohort that she followed from birth, and she graciously permitted us to bring those individuals to the lab once they were adolescents and put them in the MRI scanner. We are just starting to see the fruit from this collaboration flourish. Hill Goldsmith is a developmental psychologist who studies childhood temperament; he has been an important collaborator on many of our developmental studies. Marsha Seltzer is the director of the Waisman Center, where our Brain Imaging Lab and the Center for Investigating Healthy Minds resides. The Waisman Center is a large interdisciplinary research center with faculty from twenty-six different departments and a focus on development, broadly defined. Marsha is a great leader and also a very close and longtime personal friend. It is truly an honor and a joy to walk into the Waisman Center each day.

In addition to all the scientists who have played such an important role in my career, there are administrative folks in my lab who have been nothing short of extraordinary. Most especially is the incredible loyal dedication of Isa Dolski, who has been with me for most of my career at Wisconsin. She is an extraordinary human being, a very hard worker, and someone I can deeply trust to do the right thing. This has made my job and my life incomparably easier. My administrative assistant, Susan Jensen, has been with me now for almost ten years, and she, too, is an amazing person who handles her work with grace and dedication. In 2009 we opened the Center for Investigating Healthy Minds, which provides an umbrella for our new work on contemplative neuroscience that I describe in chapters 9 and 10. Bonnie Thorne, Mel Charbonneau, and our new executive director, Barb Mathison, have all been amazing and have helped to make this dream take shape and emerge into reality. Our Strategic Advisory Board, chaired by our lead donor, Ulco Visser, and including Steve Arnold and Jim Walsh, has provided critical advice, so needed particularly at this early stage in our development. Our Scholarly Advisory Board—Thupden Jinpa (His Holiness the Dalai Lama's translator), David Meyer, of the University of Michigan, and John Dunne, of Emory University—has provided extremely helpful feedback along the way and helped to save us from some embarrassing mistakes. John, who is Buddhist scholar extraordinaire, has been a key collaborator on a number of our meditation projects and provides a perspective from contemplative scholarship that I have come to view as not just a luxury but a real necessity for this work to proceed.

There is the concept of Sangha in some of the contemplative traditions, which means a "community" of like-minded or like-hearted individuals. I have been blessed with an extended Sangha largely due to the amazing work of the Mind and Life Institute, a nonprofit organization on whose Board of Directors I sit, whose mission is the promotion of a dialogue between Western science and the contemplative traditions, particularly Buddhism. It is in part through service to this organization that I have such frequent contact with two of my close friends, Dan Goleman and Jon Kabat-Zinn, both of whom I first met in the early 1970s. I first met Matthieu Ricard through Mind and Life, and he has become an extremely close friend and teacher. Adam Engle, the founder and chairman of the board of Mind and Life, has been a close friend for decades and has played such an important role in catalyzing the development of contemplative neuroscience.

As I describe throughout the book, my own meditation practice has been an important part of my life for more than thirty-five years. There are many people who have nurtured this part of me, beginning with my first teacher, Goenka, in 1974. Since then I have had a number of other influential teachers, including Joseph Goldstein, Jack Kornfield, Sharon Salzberg, Mingyur Rinpoche, and His Holiness the Dalai Lama. The Dalai Lama has played a monumental role in my life that I could never have imagined. I first met him in 1992 and have had the honor and privilege of seeing him on several occasions each year since. He inspires me in so many ways and has helped me to focus much of my current work on healthy qualities of mind.

My research would not have been possible without the generous support of many agencies. The University of Wisconsin, Madison, has provided a supportive home for my work since I first moved here in 1985. My family and I have come to love Madison. The National Institutes of Health (NIH) has provided continuous support to me for more than thirty years. Most of this support has come from the National Institute of Mental Health. More recently, I have also received support from the National Center for Complementary and Alternative Medicine, the National Institute on Aging, and the National Institute for Child Health and Human Development, now known as the Eunice

Kennedy Shriver National Institute for Child Health and Human Development. In addition to the NIH, I have received support from many private foundations over the years, the most significant of which have been the John D. and Catherine T. MacArthur Foundation and the Fetzer Institute.

This book has been a very long time in the making. The first real catalyst for the book was my agent, Linda Loewenthal. Linda really believed in me and hung in there with me during periods when I had noble intentions but was so consumed by ongoing research work that the thought of writing a book was daunting. Linda helped me to see that a coauthor was a possible way to proceed, and I am so lucky and honored to have connected with Sharon Begley. Linda helped to facilitate this partnership, and for this and so much else I am so grateful. Caroline Sutton, at Hudson Street Press, has provided extremely important editorial suggestions, asking wonderful and direct questions that have helped to improve the clarity in many places.

Finally, I want to thank my dear family, to whom I am so extraordinarily grateful. I have a wonderful wife, who lives her life in an inspiring way and exemplifies compassion in action. She has taught and continues to teach me so much. My children, Amelie and Seth, have also been incredible teachers and have accompanied me on so many parts of this journey. For their love and support I am so deeply grateful. And finally my mom: She is eighty-six at this writing and has been a wonderful champion of my work. Thank you, Mom, for all that you have done to enable me to do what I do today.

If this book helps you to become a little bit more aware of your Emotional Style, then it will have served its purpose. From this awareness can arise the intention to transform, if that is what you wish. May you, the readers of this book, benefit from whatever insights you may glean from this book and flourish in your well-being.

Richard Davidson
Madison, Wisconsin, June 26, 2011

NOTES

Introduction

ix **My thirty years of research in affective neuroscience:** R. J. Davidson, "Affective Style, Psychopathology, and Resilience: Brain Mechanisms and Plasticity," *American Psychologist* 55 (2000): 1196–214; R. J. Davidson, "Affective Neuroscience and Psychophysiology. Toward a Synthesis," *Psychophysiology* 40 (2003): 655–65.

x **director of the university's Center for Investigating Healthy Minds:** See www.investigatinghealthyminds.org.

xi **emotional states, emotional traits, personality, and temperament:** P. Ekman and R. J. Davidson, eds., *The Nature of Emotion: Fundamental Questions* (New York: Oxford University Press, 1994).

xi **Emotional *Style* is a consistent way of responding to the experiences of our lives:** R. J. Davidson, "Affective Style and Affective Disorders: Perspectives from Affective Neuroscience," *Cognition and Emotion* 12 (1998): 307–30.

Chapter 1

2 **One important example of this:** T. Li, L. A. Lange, X. Li, L. Susswein, B. Bryant, R. Malone, E. M. Lange, T.-Y. Huang, D. W. Stafford, and J. P. Evans, "Polymorphisms in the *VKORC1* Gene Are Strongly Associated with Warfarin Dosage Requirements in Patients Receiving Anticoagulation," *Journal of Medical Genetics* 43 (2006): 740–44.

9 **in which you have expertise:** I. Gauthier, M. J. Tarr, A. W. Anderson, P. Skudlarski, and J. C. Gore, "Activation of the Middle Fusiform 'Face Area' Increases with Expertise in Recognizing Novel Objects," *Nature Neuroscience* 2 (1999): 568–73.

9   **In fact, this fusiform gyrus:** N. Kanwisher, J. McDermott, and M. M. Chun, "The Fusiform Face Area: A Module in Human Extrastriate Cortex Specialized for Face Perception," *Journal of Neuroscience* 17 (1997): 4302–11.

9   **The brains of virtuoso violinists:** T. Elbert, C. Pantev, C. Weinbruch, B. Rockstroh, and E. Taub, "Increased Cortical Representation of the Fingers of the Left Hand in String Players," *Science* 270 (1995): 305–7.

9   **and the brains of London taxicab drivers:** E. A. Maguire, K. Woollett, and H. J. Spiers, "London Taxi Drivers and Bus Drivers: A Structural MRI and Neuropsychological Analysis," *Hippocampus* 16 (2006): 1091–1101.

10   **Scientists led by Alvaro Pascual-Leone:** A. Pascual-Leone, A. Amedi, F. Fregni, and L. B. Merabet, "The Plastic Human Brain Cortex," *Annual Review of Neuroscience* 28 (2005): 377–401.

Chapter 2

13   **Some of the most prominent researchers in psychology declared:** H. A. Simon, "Motivational and Emotional Controls of Cognition," *Psychology Review* 74 (1967): 29–39.

15   **Darwin also dabbled in human and animal emotion:** C. A. Darwin, *The Expression of the Emotions in Man and Animals* (London: Murray, 1872).

15   **In the 1970s, a handful of psychologists continued in this tradition:** P. Ekman, E. R. Sorenson, and W. V. Friesen, "Pan-Cultural Elements in Facial Displays of Emotion," *Science* 164 (1969): 86–88; S. W. Hiatt, J. J. Campos, and R. N. Emde, "Facial Patterning and Infant Emotional Expression: Happiness, Surprise, and Fear," *Child Development* 50 (1979): 1020–35.

17   **emotion comprises dual fundamental constituents:** S. Schachter and J. E. Singer, "Cognitive, Social, and Physiological Determinants of Emotional State," *Psychological Review* 69 (1962): 379–99.

21   **Perhaps the best-known example was Phineas Gage:** H. Damasio, T. Grabowski, R. Frank, A. M. Galaburda, and A. R. Damasio, "The Return of Phineas Gage: Clues About the Brain from the Skull of a Famous Patient," *Science* 264 (1994): 1102–5.

23   **In it I found a paper by an Italian neurologist at the University of Perugia named Guido Gainotti:** G. Gainotti, "Emotional Behavior and Hemispheric Side of the Lesion," *Cortex* 8 (1972): 41–55.

25   **I published the paper in the prestigious journal *Science:*** G. E. Schwartz, R. J. Davidson, and F. Maer, "Right Hemisphere Lateralization for Emotion in the Human Brain: Interactions with Cognition," *Science* 190 (1975): 286–88.

27   **Thank God our electrodes picked up activity in the visual cortex:** R. J. Davidson, G. E. Schwartz, and L. P. Rothman, "Attentional Style and the Self-Regulation of Mode-Specific Attention: An EEG Study," *Journal of Abnormal Psychology* 85 (1976): 611–21.

27   **This was the first published study in which EEGs had detected people's interior emotional states:** R. J. Davidson and G. E. Schwartz, "Patterns

of Cerebral Lateralization During Cardiac Biofeedback Versus the Self-Regulation of Emotion: Sex Differences," *Psychophysiology* 13 (1976): 62–68.

34 **Only when both muscle groups participated did we see a shift toward greater left-side activation in the brain:** P. Ekman, R. J. Davidson, and W. V. Friesen, "The Duchenne Smile: Emotional Expression and Brain Physiology II," *Journal of Personality and Social Psychology* 58 (1990): 342–53.

36 **The study was published in *Science*, and with this, the field of affective neuroscience—the study of the brain basis of emotion—was launched:** R. J. Davidson and N. A. Fox, "Asymmetrical Brain Activity Discriminates Between Positive Versus Negative Affective Stimuli in Human Infants," *Science* 218 (1982): 1235–37.

37 **Even though the prefrontal cortex is still very immature at birth, it shows functional differences associated with positive and negative emotions right from the start:** N. A. Fox and R. J. Davidson, "Taste-Elicited Changes in Facial Signs of Emotion and the Asymmetry of Brain Electrical Activity in Human Newborns," *Neuropsychologia* 24 (1986): 417–22.

38 **The measures of baseline brain activity predicted these responses perfectly:** R. J. Davidson and N. A. Fox, "Frontal Brain Asymmetry Predicts Infants' Response to Maternal Separation," *Journal of Abnormal Psychology* 98 (1989): 127–31.

39 **Presto: Individuals with depressive symptoms had significantly less activation in the left frontal region compared with nondepressed participants:** C. E. Schaffer, R. J. Davidson, and C. Saron, "Frontal and Parietal Electroencephalogram Asymmetry in Depressed and Nondepressed Subjects," *Biological Psychiatry* 18 (1983): 753–62.

39 **In fact, the great comparative psychologist T. C. Schneirla:** T. C. Schneirla, "An Evolutionary and Developmental Theory of Biphasic Processes Underlying Approach and Withdrawal," in *Nebraska Symposium on Motivation, 1959*, M. R. Jones, ed. (Oxford: University of Nebraska Press, 1959), 1–42.

40 **But it was only in 1989, when I was reviewing the raw data from those studies for a book chapter:** R. J. Davidson and A. J. Tomarken, "Laterality and Emotion: An Electrophysiological Approach," in *Handbook of Neuropsychology*, F. Boller and J. Grafman, eds. (Amsterdam, Netherlands: Elsevier, 1989), 419–41.

Chapter 3

45 **The blink reflex relates to recovery from an emotional setback:** S. K. Sutton, R. J. Davidson, B. Donzella, W. Irwin, and D. A. Dottl, "Manipulating Affective State Using Extended Picture Presentation," *Psychophysiology* 34 (1997): 217–26.

45 **We can use this fact to track what happens in the time after someone has looked at the upsetting photos:** D. C. Jackson, C. J. Mueller, I. V. Dolski, K. M. Dalton, J. B. Nitschke, H. L. Urry, M. A. Rosenkranz, C. D. Ryff, B. H. Singer,

and R. J. Davidson, "Now You Feel It, Now You Don't: Frontal Brain Electrical Asymmetry and Individual Differences in Emotion Regulation," *Psychological Science* 14 (2003): 612–17.

49 **In people who fall at the Positive extreme, brain circuits associated with positive emotion stay active for much longer:** A. S. Heller, T. Johnstone, A. J. Shackman, S. Light, M. Peterson, G. Kolden, N. Kalin, and R. J. Davidson, "Reduced Capacity to Sustain Positive Emotion in Major Depression Reflects Diminished Maintenance of Fronto-Striatal Brain Activation," *Proceedings of the National Academy of Sciences* 106 (2009): 22445–50.

52 **In the lab, we assess Social Intuition through measurements of both brain function and behavior:** K. M. Dalton, B. M. Nacewicz, T. Johnstone, H. S. Shaefer, M. A. Gernsbacher, H. H. Goldsmith, A. L. Alexander, and R. J. Davidson, "Gaze Fixation and the Neural Circuitry of Face Processing in Autism," *Nature Neuroscience* 8 (2005): 519–26.

55 **In the lab, one way we measure people's sensitivity to their internal physiological signals is by how well they can detect their own heartbeat:** R. J. Davidson, M. E. Horowitz, G. E. Schwartz, and D. M. Goodman, "Lateral Differences in the Latency Between Finger Tapping and the Heartbeat," *Psychophysiology* 18 (1981): 36–41; S. S. Khalsa, D. Rudrauf, A. R. Damasio, R. J. Davidson, A. Lutz, and D. Tranel, "Interoceptive Awareness in Experienced Meditators," *Psychophysiology* 45 (2008): 671–77.

57 **In the lab, we measure this dimension by determining how emotional behavior varies with social context:** R. J. Davidson, D. C. Jackson, and N. H. Kalin, "Emotion, Plasticity, Context, and Regulation: Perspectives from Affective Neuroscience," *Psychological Bulletin* 126 (2000): 890–909.

60 **One is selective attention:** A. Lutz, H. Slagter, N. Rawlings, A. Francis, L. L. Greischar, and R. J. Davidson, "Mental Training Enhances Attentional Stability: Neural and Behavioral Evidence," *Journal of Neuroscience* 29 (2009): 13418–27.

61 **To measure open, nonjudgmental awareness in the lab, we start with the fact that if one stimulus hijacks our attention:** H. A. Slagter, A. Lutz, L. L. Greischar, A. D. Francis, S. Nieuwenhuis, J. M. Davis, and R. J. Davidson, "Mental Training Affects Distribution of Limited Brain Resources," *PLoS Biology* 5 (2007): e138.

Chapter 4

69 **Once I was at Madison, I therefore began to reflect more deeply on what the variations in patterns of prefrontal function might mean:** R. J. Davidson, "What Does the Prefrontal Cortex 'Do' in Affect: Perspectives in Frontal EEG Asymmetry Research," *Biological Psychology* 67 (2004): 219–34.

69 **To test this idea, graduate student Daren Jackson and I recruited forty-seven adults with an average age of fifty-eight:** Jackson et al., "Now You Feel It, Now You Don't."

72 **Thanks to MRI we now know that the more white matter (axons that**

connect one neuron to another) lying between the prefrontal cortex
and the amygdala: M. J. Kim and P. J. Whalen, "The Structural Integrity of an
Amygdala-Prefrontal Pathway Predicts Trait Anxiety," *Journal of Neuroscience* 29
(2009): 11614–18.

74 Since we published this account of the autistic brain in 2005: Dalton et
al., "Gaze Fixation."

74 Moreover, the faithful and romantically committed prairie vole has
abundant oxytocin receptors in its brain, while the feckless and unattached montane vole does not: L. J. Young, Z. Wang, and T. R. Insel, "Neuroendocrine Bases of Monogamy," *Trends in Neurosciences* 21 (1998): 71–75.

74 In people, too, oxytocin has been linked to maternal behavior (it is
released during childbirth and breast-feeding), romantic attachment,
and feelings of calm and contentment: T. R. Insel, "The Challenge of Translation in Social Neuroscience: A Review of Oxytocin, Vasopressin, and Affiliative
Behavior," *Neuron* 65 (2010): 768–79.

74 But in any case, experiments with oxytocin have confirmed the role of
the amygdala in the social brain: I. Labuschagne, K. L. Phan, A. Wood, M.
Angstadt, P. Chua, M. Heinrichs, J. C. Stout, and P. J. Nathan, "Oxytocin Attenuates Amygdala Reactivity to Fear in Generalized Social Anxiety Disorder," *Neuro-
psychopharmacology* 35 (2010): 2403–13.

75 Out of a hundred monkeys shown human profiles, we identified fifteen who stayed frozen much longer than the others: Davidson et al.,
"Emotion, Plasticity, Context, and Regulation."

76 But in a recent study of rhesus monkeys with Kalin: J. A. Oler, A. S. Fox,
S. E. Shelton, J. Rogers, T. D. Dyer, R. J. Davidson, W. Shelledy, T. R. Oakes, J.
Blangero, and N. H. Kalin, "Amygdalar and Hippocampal Substrates of Anxious
Temperament Differ in Their Heritability," *Nature* 466 (2010): 864–68.

78 There is now an abundance of research, in both people and lab animals, implicating the hippocampus: C. Ranganath, "A Unified Framework
for the Functional Organization of the Medial Temporal Lobes and the Phenom-
enology of Episodic Memory," *Hippocampus* 20 (2010): 1263–90.

78 Back in graduate school, I began to study a personality type characterized by what was then called repressive defensiveness: D. A. Wein-
berger, G. E. Schwartz, and R. J. Davidson, "Low-Anxious, High-Anxious, and
Repressive Coping Styles: Psychometric Patterns and Behavioral and Physiological Responses to Stress," *Journal of Abnormal Psychology* 88 (1979): 369–80.

79 A key region of the brain for self-awareness is the insula: A. D. Craig,
"Human Feelings: Why Are Some More Aware Than Others?" *Trends in Cognitive
Sciences* 8 (2004): 239–41; A. D. Craig, "How Do You Feel? Interoception: The Sense
of the Physiological Condition of the Body," *Nature Reviews Neuroscience* 3 (2002):
655–66.

80 British researchers have found through neuroimaging: H. D. Critchley, S.
Wiens, P. Rotshtein, A. Ohman, and R. J. Dolan, "Neural Systems Supporting Interoceptive Awareness," *Nature Neuroscience* 7 (2004): 189–95.

80 In a 2010 study, also in Britain, scientists had people answer ques-
    tions designed to assess where they fall on a scale of alexithymia: G.
    Bird, G. Silani, R. Brindley, S. White, U. Frith, and T. Singer, "Empathic Brain Re-
    sponses in Insula Are Modulated by Levels of Alexithymia but Not Autism,"
    Brain 133 (2010): 1515–25.

81 In 2007, I sat down with Aaron Heller, a terrifically talented graduate
    student who had joined my lab in 2005: Heller et al., "Reduced Capacity to
    Sustain Positive Emotion."

85 Recent findings in laboratory rodents suggest that the dopamine ac-
    tivity in the nucleus accumbens may be associated with the motiva-
    tional component of reward, which underlies drive and persistence,
    while the endogenous opiates in the nucleus accumbens may be more
    associated with feelings of pleasure: M. L. Kringelbach and K. C. Berridge,
    "Towards a Functional Neuroanatomy of Pleasure and Happiness," *Trends in
    Cognitive Sciences* 13 (2009): 479–87.

85 When the opiate receptors in the nucleus accumbens are activated,
    they stimulate an adjacent brain region, the ventral pallidum: K. S.
    Smith, K. C. Berridge, and J. W. Aldridge, "Disentangling Pleasure from Incentive
    Salience and Learning Signals in Brain Reward Circuitry," *Proceedings of the Na-
    tional Academy of Sciences* 108 (2011): E255–64.

86 Humans have the capacity to focus attention through two related
    mechanisms: A. Lutz, H. A. Slagter, J. D. Dunne, and R. J. Davidson, "Attention
    Regulation and Monitoring in Meditation," *Trends in Cognitive Sciences* 12 (2008):
    163–69.

87 After giving the Tellegen questionnaire to 150 Harvard undergradu-
    ates, whom you'd expect to be a highly focused bunch: R. J. Davidson,
    G. E. Schwartz, and L. P. Rothman, "Attentional Style and the Self-Regulation of
    Mode-Specific Attention: An Electroencephalographic Study," *Journal of Abnor-
    mal Psychology* 85 (1976): 611–21.

87 With this as our guide, we did an experiment in which we fitted par-
    ticipants with headphones: Lutz et al., "Mental Training Enhances Atten-
    tional Stability."

88 Open, nonjudgmental awareness also arises from specific patterns of
    brain activity: Ibid.

Chapter 5

91 After all, a newborn has not had any life experiences that could influ-
    ence her Emotional Style: K. J. Saudino, "Behavioral Genetics and Child Tem-
    perament," *Journal of Developmental and Behavioral Pediatrics* 26 (2005): 214–23.

92 *It may well have an effect on emotions, personality, and temperament,
    but if so, that has yet to be shown: L. Thompson, J. Kemp, P. Wilson, R. Pritch-
    ett, H. Minnis, L. Toms-Whittle, C. Puckering, J. Law, and C. Gillberg, "What Have
    Birth Cohort Studies Asked About Genetic, Pre- and Perinatal Exposures and Child

and Adolescent Onset Mental Health Outcomes? A Systematic Review," *European Child and Adolescent Psychiatry* 19 (2010): 1–15.

92 **And indeed, studies comparing identical twins with fraternal ones have produced compelling evidence that genes push us to be shy or bold, risk-taking or cautious, happy or unhappy, anxious or mellow, focused or scattered:** C. A.Van Hulle, K. S. Lemery, and H. H. Goldsmith, "Wisconsin Twin Panel," *Twin Research* 5 (2002): 502–5.

93 **Even in traits with some genetic component, genes are not everything:** K. L. Kopnisky, W. M. Cowan, and S. E. Hyman, "Levels of Analysis in Psychiatric Research," *Development and Psychopathology* 14 (2002): 437–61.

94 **Kagan pioneered the study of behavioral inhibition:** J. Kagan, J. S. Reznick, and J. Gibbons, "Inhibited and Uninhibited Types of Children," *Child Development* 60 (1989): 838–45.

94 **His major finding came from a years-long study of scores of children:** C. E. Schwartz, C. I. Wright, L. M. Shin, J. Kagan, and S. L. Rauch, "Inhibited and Uninhibited Infants 'Grown Up': Adult Amygdalar Response to Novelty," *Science* 300 (2003): 1952–53.

96 **But then came a remarkable study:** A. Caspi, J. McClay, T. E. Moffitt, J. Mill, J. Martin, I. W. Craig, A. Taylor, and R. Poulton, "Role of Genotype in the Cycle of Violence in Maltreated Children," *Science* 297 (2002): 851–54.

97 **The scientists followed up this study by looking at the same New Zealanders to see whether a similar nature-nurture dance was going on with another gene:** A. Caspi, K. Sugden, T. E. Moffitt, A. Taylor, I. W. Craig, H. Harrington, J. McClay, et al., "Influence of Life Stress on Depression: Moderation by a Polymorphism in the 5-HTT Gene," *Science* 301 (2003): 386–89. This is a controversial finding, and there have been several failures to replicate it, including failures in large meta-analyses. For reviews on both sides of the debate, see M. R. Munafò, C. Durrant, G. Lewis, and J. Flint, "Gene X Environment Interactions at the Serotonin Transporter Locus," *Biological Psychiatry* 65 (2009): 211–19; N. Risch, R. Herrell, T. Lehner, K. Y. Liang, L. Eaves, J. Hoh, A. Griem, M. Kovacs, J. Ott, and K. R. Merikangas, "Interaction Between the Serotonin Transporter Gene (5-HTTLPR), Stressful Life Events, and Risk of Depression: A Meta-Analysis," *JAMA* 301 (2009): 2462–71; A. Caspi, A. R. Hariri, A. Holmes, R. Uher, and T. E. Moffitt, "Genetic Sensitivity to the Environment: The Case of the Serotonin Transporter Gene and Its Implications for Studying Complex Diseases and Traits," *American Journal of Psychiatry* 167 (2010): 509–27.

98 **The reason some rats shrug off stressful experiences so nonchalantly, Meaney and his colleagues discovered in 1989:** M. J. Meaney, S. Bhatnagar, S. Larocque, C. McCormick, N. Shanks, S. Sharma, J. Smythe, V. Viau, and P. M. Plotsky, "Individual Differences in the Hypothalamic-Pituitary-Adrenal Stress Response and the Hypothalamic CRF System," *Annals of the New York Academy of Sciences* 697 (1993): 70–85.

98 **In the mid-1990s Meaney discovered that the reason some rats had more glucocorticoid receptors in their brains:** T. Y. Zhang and M. J.

Meaney, "Epigenetics and the Environmental Regulation of the Genome and Its Function," *Annual Review of Psychology* 61 (2010): 439–66.

100 **Meaney found more sympathetic editors at *Nature Neuroscience:***I. C. Weaver, N. Cervoni, F. A. Champagne, A. C. D'Alessio, S. Sharma, J. R. Seckl, S. Dymov, M. Szyf, and M. J. Meaney, "Epigenetic Programming by Maternal Behavior," *Nature Neuroscience* 7 (2004): 847–54.

100 **Meaney studied samples from thirty-six brains:** P. O. McGowan, A. Sasaki, A. C. D'Alessio, S. Dymov, B. Labonté, M. Szyf, G. Turecki, and M. J. Meaney, "Epigenetic Regulation of the Glucocorticoid Receptor in Human Brain Associates with Childhood Abuse," *Nature Neuroscience* 12 (2009): 342–48.

101 **A 2005 study showed how important experiences are for this:** M. F. Fraga, E. Ballestar, M. F. Paz, S. Ropero, F. Setien, M. L. Ballestar, D. Heine-Suñer, et al., "Epigenetic Differences Arise During the Lifetime of Monozygotic Twins," *Proceedings of the National Academy of Sciences* 102 (2005): 10604–9.

108 **The fact that the correlation between behavioral inhibition at age three and behavioral inhibition at age nine was .03:** R. J. Davidson and M. D. Rickman, "Behavioral Inhibition and the Emotional Circuitry of the Brain: Stability and Plasticity During the Early Childhood Years," in *Extreme Fear, Shyness, and Social Phobia: Origins, Biological Mechanisms, and Clinical Outcomes*, L. A. Schmidt and J. Schulkin, eds. (New York: Oxford University Press, 1999), 67–87.

Chapter 6

114 **The world's first physicians—men such as the Greek anatomists Erasistratus in the third century BC, Galen (Marcus Aurelius's doctor) in the second century:** M. M. Mesulam and J. Perry, "The Diagnosis of Love-Sickness: Experimental Psychophysiology Without the Polygraph," *Psychophysiology* 9 (1972): 546–51.

117 **In 2005, when two prominent health psychologists counted the studies of depression and health:** S. D. Pressman and S. Cohen, "Does Positive Affect Influence Health?" *Psychological Bulletin* 131 (2005): 925–71.

118 **Fortunately, psychologist Daniel Kahneman figured out that you can't trust people to honestly and accurately tell you how satisfied or happy they are with their lives:** D. Kahneman, A. B. Krueger, D. A. Schkade, N. Schwarz, and A. A. Stone, "A Survey Method for Characterizing Daily Life Experience: The Day Reconstruction Method," *Science* 306 (2004): 1776–80.

120 **In one, Andrew Steptoe and Michael Marmot, of University College London:** A. Steptoe, J. Wardle, and M. Marmot, "Positive Affect and Health-Related Neuroendocrine, Cardiovascular, and Inflammatory Processes," *Proceedings of the National Academy of Sciences* 102 (2005): 6508–12.

121 **In one of the most convincing studies of this, health psychologist Sheldon Cohen, of Carnegie Mellon University:** S. Cohen, W. J. Doyle, R. B. Turner, C. M. Alper, and D. P. Skoner, "Emotional Style and Susceptibility to the Common Cold," *Psychosomatic Medicine* 65 (2003): 652–57.

122 **One enterprising team got their hands on journal entries, letters, and other autobiographical writings made by a group of young nuns:** D. D. Danner, D. A. Snowdon, and W. V. Friesen, "Positive Emotions in Early Life and Longevity: Findings from the Nun Study," *Journal of Personality and Social Psychology* 80 (2001): 804–13.

122 **Another excellent study followed sixty-five- to ninety-nine-year-old Mexican Americans for two years:** G. V. Ostir, K. S. Markides, S. A. Black, and J. S. Goodwin, "Emotional Well-Being Predicts Subsequent Functional Independence and Survival," *Journal of the American Geriatrics Society* 48 (2000): 473–78.

123 **Also impressive is a 2001 study that measured positive emotions in healthy seniors:** G. V. Ostir, K. S. Markides, M. K. Peek, and J. S. Goodwin, "The Association Between Emotional Well-Being and the Incidence of Stroke in Older Adults," *Psychosomatic Medicine* 63 (2001): 210–15.

123 **In a convincing 2008 review of seventy studies in both ill and healthy people:** Y. Chida and A. Steptoe, "Positive Psychological Well-Being and Mortality: A Quantitative Review of Prospective Observational Studies," *Psychosomatic Medicine* 70 (2008): 741–56.

126 **I teamed up with a Madison colleague, psychology professor Arthur Glenberg, and his graduate student David Havas:** D. A. Havas, A. M. Glenberg, K. A. Gutowski, M. J. Lucarelli, and R. J. Davidson, "Cosmetic Use of Botulinum Toxin-A Affects Processing of Emotional Language," *Psychological Science* 21 (2010): 895–900.

128 **In his earlier asthma study, William had teamed up with psychologist Chris Coe, who studies psychoneuroimmunology:** L. Y. Liu, C. L. Coe, C. A. Swenson, E. A. Kelly, H. Kita, and W. W. Busse, "School Examinations Enhance Airway Inflammation to Antigen Challenge," *American Journal of Respiratory and Critical Care Medicine* 165 (2002): 1062–67.

130 **For our first asthma study, we recruited six patients from the Madison area:** M. A. Rosenkranz, W. W. Busse, T. Johnstone, C. A. Swenson, G. M. Crisafi, M. M. Jackson, J. A. Bosch, J. F. Sheridan, and R. J. Davidson, "Neural Circuitry Underlying the Interaction Between Emotion and Asthma Symptom Exacerbation," *Proceedings of the National Academy of Sciences* 102 (2005): 13319–24.

130 **Melissa Rosenkranz, a talented graduate student, took the lead:** M. A. Rosenkranz and R. J. Davidson, "Affective Neural Circuitry and Mind-Body Influences in Asthma," *NeuroImage* 47 (2009): 972–80.

132 **I therefore got back in touch with twenty undergraduates who had participated in some of my earlier studies and had been found to have dramatically lopsided frontal activity:** D. H. Kang, R. J. Davidson, C. L. Coe, R. E. Wheeler, A. J. Tomarken, and W. B. Ershler, "Frontal Brain Asymmetry and Immune Function," *Behavioral Neuroscience* 105 (1991): 860–69.

133 **Since twenty is a fairly small number of participants, I repeated this study several years later:** R. J. Davidson, C. L. Coe, I. Dolski, and B. Donzella, "Individual Differences in Prefrontal Activation Asymmetry Predict Natural Killer

Cell Activity at Rest and in Response to Challenge," *Brain, Behavior, and Immunity* 13 (1999): 93–108.

133 **I wanted to test a more clearly valid measure of immune function, and in 2003 I realized that testing how people respond to a vaccine:** M. A. Rosenkranz, D. C. Jackson, K. M. Dalton, I. Dolski, C. D. Ryff, B. H. Singer, D. Muller, N. H. Kalin, and R. J. Davidson, "Affective Style and *In Vivo* Immune Response: Neurobehavioral Mechanisms," *Proceedings of the National Academy of Sciences* 100 (2003): 11148–52.

135 **For the experiment, I used what's called in the trade the "threat of shock" procedure more than actual shocks:** K. M. Dalton, N. H. Kalin, T. M. Grist, and R. J. Davidson, "Neural-Cardiac Coupling in Threat-Evoked Anxiety," *Journal of Cognitive Neuroscience* 17 (2005): 969–80.

Chapter 7

140 **A number of psychiatric disorders involve abnormalities in the capacity to experience pleasure:** P. E. Meehl, "Hedonic Capacity: Some Conjectures," *Bulletin of the Menninger Clinic* 39 (1975): 295–307.

142 **These were the studies in which we found that true happiness, as determined by eye-crinkling smiles:** Ekman et al., "The Duchenne Smile."

143 **Several studies had concluded that children with autism may have a fundamental abnormality in the fusiform gyrus:** R. T. Schultz, D. J. Grelotti, A. Klin, J. Kleinman, C. Van der Gaag, R. Marois, and P. Skudlarski, "The Role of the Fusiform Face Area in Social Cognition: Implications for the Pathobiology of Autism," *Philosophical Transactions of the Royal Society B: Biological Sciences* 358 (2003): 415–27.

144 **To see if my suspicion was right, my colleagues and I launched the first study:** Dalton et al., "Gaze Fixation."

146 **Among identical twins, who have identical DNA sequences, if one twin has autism, then the other does in 63 to 98 percent of the cases:** C. M. Freitag, W. Staal, S. M. Klauck, E. Duketis, and R. Waltes, "Genetics of Autistic Disorders: Review and Clinical Implications," *European Child and Adolescent Psychiatry* 19 (2010): 169–78.

147 **To see if this is so, we conducted a study of the siblings of children with autism:** Dalton et al., "Gaze Fixation."

148 **It turns out that there are almost as many species of depression as there are of beetles:** R. J. Davidson, D. Pizzagalli, J. B. Nitschke, and K. M. Putnam, "Depression: Perspectives from Affective Neuroscience," *Annual Review of Psychology* 53 (2002): 545–74.

150 **In one of my earliest studies, described in chapter 4, we showed depressed patients and healthy controls one- to two-minute clips:** R. J. Davidson, C. E. Schaffer, and C. Saron, "Effects of Lateralized Presentations of Faces on Self-Reports of Emotion and EEG Asymmetry in Depressed and Non-Depressed Subjects," *Psychophysiology* 22 (1985): 353–64.

151 **In a recent experiment, mentioned in chapter 4, we trained depressed patients and healthy controls to perform what's called cognitive reappraisal:** Heller et al., "Reduced Capacity to Sustain Positive Emotion."

154 **People with higher left than right prefrontal activity feel a greater sense of well-being and contentment:** H. L. Urry, J. B. Nitschke, I. Dolski, D. C. Jackson, K. M. Dalton, C. J. Mueller, M. A. Rosenkranz, C. D. Ryff, B. H. Singer, and R. J. Davidson, "Making a Life Worth Living: Neural Correlates of Well-Being," *Psychological Science* 15 (2004): 367–72.

155 **People who have greater baseline levels of right prefrontal activation score high on behavioral inhibition:** S. K. Sutton and R. J. Davidson, "Prefrontal Brain Asymmetry: A Biological Substrate of the Behavioral Approach and Inhibition Systems," *Psychological Science* 8 (1997): 204–10.

155 **In a large randomized control trial, 188 patients with major depressive disorder:** K. S. Dobson, S. D. Hollon, S. Dimidjian, K. B. Schmaling, R. J. Kohlenberg, R. J. Gallop, S. L. Rizvi, J. K. Gollan, D. L. Dunner, and N. S. Jacobson, "Randomized Trial of Behavioral Activation, Cognitive Therapy, and Antidepressant Medication in the Prevention of Relapse and Recurrence in Major Depression," *Journal of Consulting and Clinical Psychology* 76 (2008): 468–77.

156 **In a 2009 study, scientists performed fMRIs before and after treatment:** G. S. Dichter, J. N. Felder, C. Petty, J. Bizzell, M. Ernst, and M. J. Smoski, "The Effects of Psychotherapy on Neural Responses to Rewards in Major Depression," *Biological Psychiatry* 66 (2009): 886–97.

158 **In an analysis of sixteen such studies involving a total of 184 people with ADHD and 186 normal controls, researchers at the New York University Child Study Center:** A. M. Kelly, D. S. Margulies, and F. X. Castellanos, "Recent Advances in Structural and Functional Brain Imaging Studies of Attention-Deficit/Hyperactivity Disorder," *Current Psychiatry Reports* 9 (2007): 401–7.

158 **Here, too, when this process goes awry, the result is ADHD:** C. Dockstader, W. Gaetz, D. Cheyne, F. Wang, F. X. Castellanos, and R. Tannock, "MEG Event-Related Desynchronization and Synchronization Deficits During Basic Somatosensory Processing in Individuals with ADHD," *Behavioral and Brain Functions* 4 (2008): 8.

159 **In one 2011 study from a team in the Netherlands:** O. Tucha, L. Tucha, G. Kaumann, S. König, K. M. Lange, D. Stasik, Z. Streather, T. Engelschalk, and K. W. Lange, "Training of Attention Functions in Children with Attention Deficit Hyperactivity Disorder," *Attention Deficit and Hyperactivity Disorders*, May 20, 2011.

Chapter 8

161 **Take experiences:** A. Pascual-Leone and F. Torres, "Plasticity of the Sensorimotor Cortex Representation of the Reading Finger in Braille Readers," *Brain* 116 (1993): 39–52; A. Pascual-Leone, A. Cammarota, E. M. Wassermann, J. P.

Brasil-Neto, L. G. Cohen, and M. Hallett, "Modulation of Motor Cortical Outputs to the Reading Hand of Braille Readers," *Annals of Neurology* 34 (1993): 33–37.

162 **Even more dramatically:** N. Sadato, A. Pascual-Leone, J. Grafman, V. Ibañez, M. P. Deiber, G. Dold, and M. Hallett, "Activation of the Primary Visual Cortex by Braille Reading in Blind Subjects," *Nature* 380 (1996): 526–28.

162 **Similarly, thought alone can increase or decrease:** L. R. Baxter Jr., J. M. Schwartz, K. S. Bergman, M. P. Szuba, B. H. Guze, J. C. Mazziotta, A. Alazraki, et al., "Caudate Glucose Metabolic Rate Changes with Both Drug and Behavior Therapy for Obsessive-Compulsive Disorder," *Archives of General Psychiatry* 49 (1992): 681–89.

162 **The idea that there is a one-to-one correspondence:** Sharon Begley, *Train Your Mind, Change Your Brain: How a New Science Reveals Our Extraordinary Potential to Transform Ourselves* (New York: Ballantine Books, 2007), 26.

163 **we got Brodmann areas:** Ibid., 27.

163 **In experiments in the 1940s and 1950s:** Ibid., 87.

164 **As a result of the discoveries:** quoted in D. H. Lowenstein and J. M. Parent, "Brain, Heal Thyself," *Science* 283 (1999): 1126–27.

164 **Then the Silver Spring monkeys came along:** Caroline Fraser, "The Raid at Silver Spring," *New Yorker*, April 19, 1993.

165 **The result of that sensory deprivation:** T. P. Pons, P. E. Garraghty, A. K. Ommaya, J. H. Kaas, E. Taub, and M. Mishkin, "Massive Cortical Reorganization After Sensory Deafferentation in Adult Macaques," *Science* 252 (1991): 1857–60.

165 **In what was called the spinning disk experiment:** M. M. Merzenich, R. J. Nelson, J. H. Kaas, M. P. Stryker, W. M. Jenkins, J. M. Zook, M. S. Cynader, and A. Schoppmann, "Variability in Hand Surface Representations in Areas 3b and 1 in Adult Owl and Squirrel Monkeys," *Journal of Comparative Neurology* 258 (1987): 281–96.

166 **When scientists, also at UCSF:** R. J. Nudo, G. W. Milliken, W. M. Jenkins, and M. M. Merzenich, "Use-Dependent Alterations of Movement Representations in Primary Motor Cortex of Adult Squirrel Monkeys," *Journal of Neuroscience* 16 (1996): 785–807.

167 **also in the *auditory* cortex:** H. J. Neville, A. Schmidt, and M. Kutas, "Altered Visual-Evoked Potentials in Congenitally Deaf Adults," *Brain Research* 266 (1983): 127–32.

167 **This rezoning has practical consequences:** D. Bavelier, A. Tomann, C. Hutton, T. Mitchell, D. Corina, G. Liu, and H. Neville, "Visual Attention to the Periphery Is Enhanced in Congenitally Deaf Individuals," *Journal of Neuroscience* 20 (2000): 1–6.

167 **In blind people who become proficient:** Sadato et al., "Activation of the Primary Visual Cortex."

167 **The brains of the blind:** B. Röder, W. Teder-Sälejärvi, A. Sterr, F. Rösler, S. A. Hillyard, and H. J. Neville, "Improved Auditory Spatial Tuning in Blind Humans," *Nature* 400 (1999): 162–66.

167 **A century before these discoveries:** William James, *Psychology: The Briefer Course* (Cambridge, MA: Harvard University Press, 1985), 17.

168 **One final example:** A. Amedi, N. Raz, P. Pianka, R. Malach, and E. Zohary, "Early 'Visual' Cortex Activation Correlates with Superior Verbal Memory Performance in the Blind," *Nature Neuroscience* 6 (2003): 758–66.

168 **And in the blind:** A. Amedi, A. Floel, S. Knecht, E. Zohary, and L. G. Cohen, "Transcranial Magnetic Stimulation of the Occipital Pole Interferes with Verbal Processing in Blind Subjects," *Nature Neuroscience* 7 (2004): 1266–70.

169 **yet after a mere five days:** A. Pascual-Leone and R. Hamilton, "The Metamodal Organization of the Brain," *Progress in Brain Research* 134 (2001): 427–45.

170 **He called the treatment:** Begley, 121.

171 **Taub found what he called:** E. Taub, G. Uswatte, D. K. King, D. Morris, J. E. Crago, and A. Chatterjee, "A Placebo-Controlled Trial of Constraint-Induced Movement Therapy for Upper Extremity After Stroke," *Stroke* 37 (2006): 1045–49.

171 **As Taub's and other studies showed:** Begley, 124–25.

171 **In the violinists:** Elbert et al., "Increased Cortical Representation."

172 **"Plasticity is an intrinsic property":** Pascual-Leone et al., "The Plastic Human Brain Cortex."

173 **In *The Heart of Buddhist Meditation:*** Nyanaponika Thera, *The Heart of Buddhist Meditation: Satipatthna: A Handbook of Mental Training Based on the Buddha's Way of Mindfulness* (York Beach, ME: Samuel Weiser, 1973), 30.

173 **In the case of his OCD patients:** Jeffrey M. Schwartz and Sharon Begley, *The Mind and the Brain: Neuroplasticity and the Power of Mental Force* (New York: Regan Books, 2002).

173 **Thinking about their thoughts in a new way:** Baxter et al., "Caudate Glucose Metabolic Rate Changes."

174 **Scientists at the University of Toronto found:** K. Goldapple, Z. Segal, C. Garson, M. Lau, P. Bieling, S. Kennedy, and H. Mayberg, "Modulation of Cortical-Limbic Pathways in Major Depression: Treatment-Specific Effects of Cognitive Behavior Therapy," *Archives of General Psychiatry* 61 (2004): 34–41.

Chapter 9

183 **In one experiment, Dan Goleman and I studied with fifty-eight people who had varying degrees of experience with meditation:** R. J. Davidson, D. J. Goleman, and G. E. Schwartz, "Attentional and Affective Concomitants of Meditation: A Cross-Sectional Study," *Journal of Abnormal Psychology* 85 (1976): 235–38.

Chapter 10

202 **This would be the first truly randomized controlled trial of MBSR:** R. J. Davidson, J. Kabat-Zinn, J. Schumacher, M. A. Rosenkranz, D. Muller, S. F. Santorelli, F. Urbanowski, A. Harrington, K. Bonus, and J. F. Sheridan, "Alterations in

Brain and Immune Function Produced by Mindfulness Meditation," *Psychosomatic Medicine* 65 (2003): 564–70.

207 **We chose to study whether this intense meditation practice had any effect on attention:** Slagter et al., "Mental Training Affects Distribution of Limited Brain Resources"; H. A. Slagter, A. Lutz, L. L. Greischar, S. Nieuwenhuis, and R. J. Davidson, "Theta Phase Synchrony and Conscious Target Perception: Impact of Intensive Mental Training," *Journal of Cognitive Neuroscience* 21 (2009): 1536–49; Lutz et al., "Mental Training Enhances Attentional Stability."

210 **An intriguing new study supports the finding that mental training can alter brain patterns:** C. E. Kerr, S. R. Jones, Q. Wan, D. L. Pritchett, R. H. Wasserman, A. Wexler, J. J. Villanueva, et al., "Effects of Mindfulness Meditation Training on Anticipatory Alpha Modulation in Primary Somatosensory Cortex," *Brain Research Bulletin* 85 (2011): 96–103.

212 **For the first study, I was interested in a phenomenon called neural synchrony:** A. Lutz, L. L. Greischar, N. B. Rawlings, M. Ricard, and R. J. Davidson, "Long-Term Meditators Self-Induce High-Amplitude Synchrony During Mental Practice," *Proceedings of the National Academy of Sciences* 101 (2004): 16369–73.

214 **Using fMRI, we pinpointed regions that were active during compassion meditation:** A. Lutz, J. A. Brefczynski-Lewis, T. Johnstone, and R. J. Davidson, "Voluntary Regulation of the Neural Circuitry of Emotion by Compassion Meditation: Effects of Expertise," *PLoS One* 3 (2008): e1897.

216 **In the study, we had to work within the confines of the MRI tube, so for the focus of concentration we decided to project a dot on a screen:** J. A. Brefczynski-Lewis, A. Lutz, H. S. Schaefer, D. B. Levinson, and R. J. Davidson, "Neural Correlates of Attentional Expertise in Long-Term Meditation Practitioners," *Proceedings of the National Academy of Sciences* 104 (2007): 11483–88.

Chapter 11

231 **Another way to strengthen connections between the prefrontal cortex and the ventral striatum is a technique called well-being therapy:** G. A. Fava and E. Tomba, "Increasing Psychological Well-Being and Resilience by Psychotherapeutic Methods," *Journal of Personality* 77 (2009): 1903–34.

237 **A 2008 study found that people who have practiced mindfulness meditation every day:** B. K. Hölzel, U. Ott, T. Gard, H. Hempel, M. Weygandt, K. Morgen, and D. Vaitl, "Investigation of Mindfulness Meditation Practitioners with Voxel-Based Morphometry," *Social Cognitive and Affective Neuroscience* 3 (2008): 55–61.

241 **A study we did in 2009 suggests why:** Lutz et al., "Mental Training Enhances Attentional Stability."

INDEX